HACK YOUR WAY TO YOUR DREAM BODY, TAKE BACK YOUR POWER, AND KEEP THE UNWANTED WEIGHT OFF!

READ THIS WHEN YOU'RE DONE DIETING

MORGANA LAKATOS-HAYWARD

READ THIS WHEN YOU'RE DONE DIETING

Hack Your Way to Your Dream Body, Take Back Your Power, and Keep the Unwanted Weight Off!

Copyright © 2024. Morgana Lakatos-Hayward. All rights reserved. No part of this publication may be reproduced, distributed, or transmitted in any form or by any means, including photocopying, recording, or other electronic or mechanical methods, without the prior written permission of the publisher, except in the case of brief quotations embodied in critical reviews and certain other noncommercial uses permitted by copyright law.

For permission requests, speaking inquiries, podcast interviews, and bulk order purchase options, email morganalh@live.ca.

This Isn't a Diet
87 Garinger Crescent
Binbrook, Ont. Canada L0R1C0
thisisntadiet.com

ISBN: 979-8-9911569-1-2

Edited by Lori Lynn Enterprises | LoriLynnEnterprises.com
Designed by Transcendent Publishing | TranscendentPublishing.com

Disclaimer: The contents of this book are for educational purposes. If unsure whether any of the information or tips are right for you, consult with your doctor or a nutritionally-informed health care professional.

"Nature has given us all the pieces required to achieve exceptional wellness and health, but has left it to us to put these pieces together."

—Diane McLaren

DEDICATION

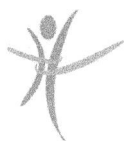

To my mom and dad, my pillar guides in this world, without whom I would not know how to stand. And to my one and only, Dominik. Without you, this book would never have come to life.

TABLE OF CONTENTS

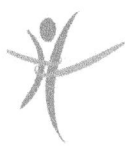

Foreword xiii

Introduction xvii
    Who This Book Is For xxii
    Who Is Morgana Lakatos-Hayward? xxiii
    What Is Women's Health? xxiv
    You Are Not Alone xxvii

CHAPTER 1 | The Real Reason Dieting Doesn't Work 1
    Risks of Processed Foods 2
    Difficult Diets 5
    Calorie Counting 6
    Liquid Diets 7
    Keto Diet 7
    Detox Diets 9
    Plant-Based 10
    The Basics 11

CHAPTER 2 | Get Your Glucose in Check 19
    Glucose Symptom Checklist 20

The Four Types of Sugars 21
Glucose Spikes 23
Insulin 29
5 Key Tips to Minimize Glucose Curves 31
Additional Small Hacks 37
Glucose Themes 39

CHAPTER 3 | Hacking Your Hormones Back into Balance 41
Hormone Symptom Checklist 42
The Endocrine System 43
Endocrine Disruptors 48
Endocrine Tips 52
Normal Problems, Normal Solutions 59
Hormonal Themes 60

CHAPTER 4 | Trust Your Gut 61
Gut-Brain Connection Symptom Checklist 62
Gut-Brain Connection Explained 63
How Are Your Emotions Involved? 74
Starting in the Womb 77
Food Addiction and Diets 79
Tips for a Happier Gut 83
Gut-Brain Themes 85

CHAPTER 5 | Eating for Energy 87
Low Energetics Symptoms Checklist 88
All About Energetics 88
Nourishing Yourself Outside of Your Plate 92
The Power to Heal Naturally 94
Oriental Medicine Beliefs 96

  Energetics Tips 101
  Energetics Themes. 103

CHAPTER 6 | A Whole New World 105

Crossing the Finish Line. 115

Acknowledgments. 117

Appendix. 119

References 123

About the Author 125

Your Free Gift 127

ADVANCE PRAISE

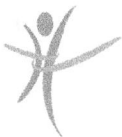

"With Morgana's program, I learned to trust my body more. Finally, (after years) I feel again more connected to my body, which is so important as a dancer, but also as a normal person. So I understand now what my body needs, when I am actually hungry, or when I am not. Now I know how to help my body when I don't feel so good. There is always a solution now.

Mentally, I am much more confident about myself. Not only about my body, but my worth and especially my 'role' as a dancer. In contrast to any other diets or lifestyle changes I tried before, I really want to keep this routine and lifestyle up because I enjoy it and it makes everything so much easier—especially because the changes are not difficult. You just need the right tools, which Morgana gave me."

—Ida-Maria Jahn

"Morgana is deeply educated, professional, and multi-talented! She is able to marry all aspects of life—physical, emotional, mental, spiritual, financial, and environmental together to work towards a focused, common goal that is created at the start of the program.

In my experience, Morgana, through her adaptability and compassionately open mindset, looked at all aspects of life to help me achieve my ultimate goal. Not many coaches would take the time to do this. Highly recommend!"

—Ava Brueske

"Morgana's program has helped me accomplish my physical and emotional goals over the course of a month and I have learned so many tips that I can implement into my busy life.

She has created such a warm and supportive environment, which helped me open up and discover what my body needs.

I have become more confident in my body, and I feel like we have constructed a sustainable plan that will improve various aspects of my life. Overall, a very positive experience!"

—Anonymous

"Working with Morgana has given me a better understanding of my body, mind, and health that I truly value. She has wonderful insight into many issues, questions, and feelings that I have been experiencing. I have now discovered a new routine for my health moving forward and I valued every conversation we had. I highly recommend this program."

—Sabrina Strasser

FOREWORD

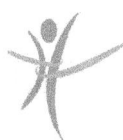

Like Morgana, I have the same stereotypical memories of being a young dancer, and I vividly remember deciding to "go on a diet" with my dancing friends at the ripe old age of ... eight!

I remember being told in quite a matter-of-fact manner, "If you lost a few kilos, you'd have less to drag around the dance floor and you'd be faster."

I thought, *Yeah, makes total sense, I'm on it!*

This was normal then. And unfortunately, it still is in some circles. Body-shaming, food-shaming, and judging each other based on a kilo here and there has become a widely accepted epidemic in the world of performers.

As if bending your body, feet, and life in ways that some may find highly unnatural wasn't enough, you also have to keep your weight, body fat percentage, and shade of tan to the exact degree stipulated by your coach. And there is certainly no negotiation on that!

But then you have people like Morgana—changing the face of health, wellness, nurturing your body, and overall fitness. Morgana and her book would have been a godsend to me back in the day when I started on my first shake diet at the tender age of 15. Shakes filled with processed chemicals and artificial sugars. Shakes with ingredients too complicated to even read. Shakes with sell by dates lasting years on end because, news flash: they're not actually food!

I would have absolutely loved my younger self to pick up a copy of *Read This When You're Done Dieting*. It would have made things a lot clearer and more reassuring.

Before even looking at Morgana's debut book, I want to explain why this lady is so extraordinary. I have never come across such a strong personification of the phrase "grit and graft." Perhaps I'm being a bit too British there, but these are the words I'd use to describe Morgana.

She is certainly one of the most determined and hardest working people I have ever had the pleasure of meeting. And this all forms part of how and why she has been able to delve so eloquently into complex themes, including nutrition basics, gut-brain connection, processed foods, and hormones.

As a nutritionist myself, I know that keeping up with the relevant updates is almost a full-time job in itself, as we are experiencing a time of rapid research. Health and wellness is a fairly new line of research for many institutions, with new findings growing in the last ten years. This is such an exciting time and shows us how much there is that we still have to learn about. This book is an excellent place to start.

Morgana and I met during a very strange time for all of us: Covid. During this time, many people decided to sit back, relax, or, alternatively, stress about the lack of opportunities we were all faced with. They let their circumstances control their outcome and life became a bit hopeless. I have zero judgment on that, especially for those with dependents—as a mother of a 2.5-year-old (and one on the way!)—I cannot even imagine how difficult that would have been.

However, Morgana absolutely flew the flag of work ethic for the entire dancing world. She grabbed life with both hands, knowing that her story did not stop at being a world-champion dancer. She had so much more to give. So much more intelligence. So much more value and love to share with the world.

She got to work and dove into building her knowledge on health, the body, how it works, how she works and how to ultimately be a happier, healthier individual. All whilst building up her financial security, maintaining high fitness levels for her dancing career and building an impressive set of social media platforms.

Morgana also cares deeply about others—she wants to share her story, advice, and tips so that other people have a less turbulent journey towards their own finish line. This is something truly unique about her: she's a badass, with a kind heart and a giving soul. A true friend.

I'd say that if you follow Morgana and her methods, you can't go far wrong with up-leveling your life across many pillars. And, of course, you should start with this book.

—Robyn Lee
Nutritionist, Author, *Positively Selfish* Podcast Host

INTRODUCTION

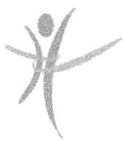

"People are fed by the food industry, which pays no attention to health, and are treated by the health industry, which pays no attention to food."

—Wendell Berry

What happened to that little girl with the big dreams and the strong work ethic? Where did she go? And what in the world is happening to my body?

As I stood there studying my reflection in the mirror, instead of feeling proud of myself for everything I had accomplished up to that point, all I could hear in my head was, "Her thighs are a bit too big."

And all I could see were the extra 5 kg (11 pounds) I couldn't seem to shake.

Before I got that critique from one of my coaches during an overseas competition, I had told myself as a young dancer that I would never give anyone the power to call me "fat."

I was always the youngest dancer in my classes, which meant I heard a lot of conversations among the "big kids." I remember hearing the older girls talk about their diets, pinch their skin, and pretend it was fat, and I would hear the whispers of teachers and parents saying, "Yes, she's good, but … she needs to lose a bit of weight."

Back then, I couldn't fathom the thought of ever going on a diet or restricting myself in any way, shape, or form. I knew about disordered eating and body perception from watching dance films. I read about it constantly in dancer interviews. But I was the ultimate chocolate lover, and restriction and bingeing never made sense to me.

Until the dreaded day finally came that put me on the same track as all the other dancers before me. Here I was, poking at my thigh and belly fat after getting up at 6 a.m. to overexercise.

I felt a deep shame and couldn't believe I'd let myself go. I took my coaches' diet advice for what worked for them, not knowing anything about my body or health knowledge in general.

I stuck to a low-carb, high-animal-protein diet without any sauces or joy. I was clinically underweight and, needless to say, hungry. My parents told me I wasn't eating enough and couldn't just eat salads every day. But what they didn't know was that I was secretly bingeing any sweets I could gather in the house when I "went to bed." It was definitely my low point.

What I would later learn is that this bingeing (shoveling loads of food in one sitting due to starvation or restriction conditions) is extremely normal in diet culture and that many other people suffer from food restriction (which is what inspired me to write this book).

Dieting can turn on your body's defense mechanism to battle self-induced famine, and your brain will eventually send out chemicals to tell your body to seek out large amounts of food for survival, hence the bingeing. This is why two-thirds of dieters regain more weight than they lost and lose tune with their bodies and bodily cues (more on this later). In my own story, I didn't know that my diet misery would get worse.

At every other competition, I would get the same feedback from different teachers that I was still "a bit too big on the thighs," or I needed to lose 5 kg. I felt hopeless. I felt like a failure to that little girl who never wanted puberty to catch up with her.

The thigh growth came in tune with my period as if one led to the other. (Only later would I learn about subcutaneous fat.) As I lost more weight, I also stopped getting my period for roughly over a year. In short, my body was confused AF.

My spirits were so low that I finally went to see a sports therapist. He gave me good advice and said he worked with many dancers and showed me statistics and the number of pounds he had helped them lose.

However, he put me on a generic, one-size-fits-all diet he used for all the athletes he worked with. He didn't run any body composition tests, completely ignoring the thought of bio-individuality (more on this soon). He emailed me his plan, telling me to eat three meals and three snacks per day and to continue doing a high-protein, low-carb diet, and he sent me on my way.

When I asked what to do when I would get my sugar cravings, he told me those were probably emotional and that I would just have to think about whether my goals were bigger than my cravings. Let me tell you, it didn't work. And it wasn't for a lack of trying. (Little did I know my adrenal fatigue, constant stress, and food addiction were fueling those cravings.) My body was fighting a war between my brain and my stomach.

One year later, still hearing the whispers behind my back about my body, I tried keto. Keto is a diet where you eat only fats and proteins and avoid carbs like the devil to put you in a state of "ketosis." This is where you burn fats as energy rather than carbs.

I was preparing for our biggest competition of the year, the Blackpool Dance Festival. I had never had such low energy levels. For the first two weeks, I remember being in training with shaking hands and feeling dizzy. I would daydream about walking into the nearby grocery store, buying a big loaf of bread, and sitting down in the parking lot, stuffing it down my throat.

After the competition was over, I was no lighter, might I add, and I cheated like never before in my life. I had carbs on top of carbs on top of carbs for two weeks straight. My acne was unheard of, and my period was only showing her face for a few months of the year.

During COVID, competitions stopped. For two straight years, I finally had the semblance of a social life and allowed myself more opportunities to feed my body. This was until I began to sell health supplements online in hopes of helping others like me and was roped into the notorious "shake diet." For one meal a day, I would have protein powder with water, and I would take all these vitamin powders and prebiotics in hopes of bettering my body and selling this miracle diet to clients.

What I didn't see coming was that what I had missed in the shake meal, I added double to my other two meals from sheer hunger pains. I gained the most amount of weight during COVID, and my periods were back and as painful as ever. My acne was out of control. I had honestly never felt so ugly.

I went to see a gynecologist who told me I had adenomyosis and that it was beginning to scar my uterus from my painful periods. He put me on birth control and, again, sent me on my way. I gained more weight, and nothing changed with my acne, only that my periods were tamed.

It was only when I had hit probably the lowest point of my life that everything changed for the better. I had broken my wrist right before a major competition in the UK and flew back home to Canada to heal at my parents' house and with my home doctors.

I had begun reading health books in my free time, and for some reason, I was taking notes (some intuitive gut feeling knew I would one day write a health book). I returned to dancing only to find out that my partner of 10 years had left me for another partner while I was recovering.

In spite of my loss, I found a new partner, and instinctively, I began eating less and less animal protein. I had always felt heavy and lethargic after meals with meat, and my health studies had started to teach me the power of plant protein. I eventually became a full vegetarian and found a healthy exercise regimen that worked for my body. I dropped the 5 kg, my acne healed, and I was happily eating carbs and meals I enjoyed.

Be that as it may, I still had so many questions that were left unanswered. Why is sugar bad? How are hormones related to other systems in the body, and how do they influence behavior and appearance? Why are we told that carbs are the enemy and salt is the devil? What on earth is gut health? And most importantly, how do all of the various bodily systems I was learning about individually affect one another and ultimately work together?

I was still confused, as I would read a book about glucose and get all these amazing tips to help manage glucose spikes. Then, I would read a book about hormones and get other tips. There was sometimes overlap, and sometimes I would see the mention of other systems or organs in play, but I needed more handholding to piece all the systems together.

This is what this book is designed to do. It is not just about gut health or glucose or hormones. It links the connections and tools you can use to heal your body once and for all and teaches you how your body systems interact. It even takes it a step further to address the energy and energetics that our foods hold and will teach you to stray away from diet culture and instead get back in tune with your beautiful body.

I am so excited to share my information with you, and I hope that it will heal whatever problem caused you to pick up this book and start reading.

So, without further ado, let's get started.

Who This Book Is For

This book is for the woman who is ready to take matters into her own hands. She's tried the whole diet culture craze and felt it didn't quite sit right with her beliefs. At her core, she knows that dieting is short-term and not sustainable. Her intuition is telling her there's a better way. And she's right.

Many health beliefs and stereotypes are targeted toward men, and many health-related scientific studies include only a small percentage of women due to the changes our systems go through during our menstruation cycle. But that's *exactly* why there needs to be more education and resources for women to break through the misinformation and learn how to heal and nourish our amazing bodies.

It is my hope that this book will help you to gain an appreciation for your beautiful body. Today, I see and work with so many women who would love to change at least 10 things about their body ASAP. Social media and the photoshopping capabilities in the media are to blame, and we usually fall victim to "comparisonitis."

If you knew everything your body does in one second, let alone a day, I think you would be amazed and want to help it do its job better (and you'll see the benefits too). I also hope that you learn to steer clear of the enticing packaging and advertising of the latest dieting craze available. I have no doubt that there will be hundreds more diets and trends developed, when really, as women, we need to get back to our roots.

When we take care of our blood sugar balance, nourish our hormones, and supercharge our gut health, we become unstoppable. You will notice yourself smashing your goals without all the headaches and hassle that diets create. Most importantly, you will be able to implement these into a *lasting* lifestyle routine you can experiment with and choose from! Ditch diet culture and the unrealistic, unattainable rules it sets, and you'll find a manageable plan that yields results.

This journey we are about to embark on is one I hope you will love and cherish, the same way I have while writing this book for you. Whoever you are and wherever you may be, we are connected through the love of bettering ourselves and making ourselves our first priority. I am so excited to share this information with you, and I hope you're just as excited about reading it.

If you feel you need more personalized support, you can reach out to me through my website at:

thisisntadiet.com

You'll find that I am more than happy to help you!

Who Is Morgana Lakatos-Hayward?

On the surface, for many years, my life might have seemed perfect. I had world championship titles in dancing, I was traveling the world from a young age, had friends in different countries, was in the gym or on the treadmill every day at 6 a.m., and was still pursuing a higher education. However, the glam and seemingly too-perfect circumstances were, in fact, a facade.

Deep down, I was so unhappy. I couldn't look into a mirror without hating what was reflected back (and I danced every day for multiple hours in front of mirrors).

I was so burnt out and emotionally and physically exhausted that when I wasn't in the studio or gym, I was sleeping. I had no semblance of an outside life. I had no idea who I was without dancing, and yet, somehow, I never felt enough in this world that put pretty girls with amazing figures on a pedestal while I struggled to maintain any sort of shape.

It was when I went in search of a better way that I began to hold appreciation for myself. It wasn't my fault I couldn't sustain a diet for more than two months! These diets are unattainable and foreign to the way our bodies are designed to function.

Funnily enough, through breaking free from restriction, learning what foods serve my body and mind, and implementing easy hacks into my lifestyle, I finally got to the shape I had always wanted.

I effortlessly dropped the 5 kg I was always struggling with. The puffiness in my face and muscles vanished, and my acne cleared. My hair started growing again, my PMS symptoms disappeared, and my uterus growth vanished. I had heaps more energy, and I was a better and happier human being overall!

And, girl, I still eat pasta, bread, chocolate, pastries, burgers, and pizza whenever my little ol' heart desires it!

I am so grateful I had beautiful, inspirational female guides leading me toward the information I needed in my life through the use of books and podcasts, which led me to attend the Institute for Integrative Nutrition (IIN), where my love of nutrition and health on a full spectrum blossomed.

Now, I hope to return some of that magic to you and give you a spark of hope on your own journey of transformation.

What Is Women's Health?

This book delves into the world of information your body holds. We start off by educating you about the basics; then we get into more complex systems that are vital to your health and well-being as a woman.

We'll discuss managing your glucose levels, explain why it's important, and cover what you can do to help this system. Then, we'll continue on to your hormones, an important topic in women's health.

We will also discuss your gut and how and why keeping it healthy will dramatically keep you and your mind in good shape, as well as helping you make better choices for your body.

Lastly, we will delve into the world of food energetics and some practices of oriental medicine, as I am a huge believer in returning to the root cause rather than just treating symptoms.

I will connect all these systems to show you how they are intertwined and dependent on one another.

So why do you need to know this?

Well, let's take a second and connect to your inner desires. I want you to list five things you would change about your body if you could. Take a second here and write it down if you want.

1. _____
2. _____
3. _____
4. _____
5. _____

For some of the self-critical gals out there, I'm sure this exercise could be done quickly, and if that's you, I'm sure you could name more than five because I used to be the same way! But let's go ahead and change the narrative.

So, let's say one of the things you wrote was:

"I want to lose 10 pounds by May."

Now, first, let's change that to gain more body appreciation but also to help you change on a cellular level:

"I am so appreciative of my body holding on to resources to keep me safe. I understand that it is a safety mechanism as I haven't been using the right practices to care for it. I am now ready to release what isn't serving me and show up as my best self."

(**Note**: In this book, you will learn how your body and mind are so connected that your cells actually listen and feel what you are thinking.)

Go ahead and reframe your beliefs. You can even create a sticky note board with these affirmations that you will see in your home. This is exactly why this book found you.

For some reason, you picked it up because, subconsciously, you were sick of feeling guilt, shame, and negativity around your body. You wanted to do right by you.

Even if you are a health expert girlie reading this, keep an open mind as you might learn a thing or two. Or, if you are starting from scratch on this journey, take what you can and leave what you don't need. It's designed to be a guide, not a gospel.

My approach to health is unique as I help women in so many areas. Many practitioners niche their expertise down so much that they fail to take into account how everything works together! I aid in the management of blood sugar and hormone balancing, as well as getting your gut healthy and working efficiently in the physical aspect.

In my work with clients, I also get into their mental and emotional blocks to tackle why they make certain decisions and to help them deal with their stress in healthier ways. This also has a dramatic impact on their lifestyle and energy levels.

This conversation can even lead to other areas of life, such as navigating financial stress and relationships, finding creative outlets, and learning to develop spiritual practices that are right for them and their beliefs. Everything is connected, and that is vital to my practice and the way I go about my life.

You've already begun your journey by reframing your beliefs. To continue, I encourage you to experiment throughout this book. See which hacks work best for you and track them.

You can do this by keeping a food journal and writing down your meals and how you feel afterward. You can also do this by taking pictures of your food and noticing patterns. Whichever way is best for you, be aware of your body.

You can't do all the hacks 100% of the time, so you should try them and feel what works for you. You are different from the next girl who picks up this book, and you are even different from me. I am allergic to strawberries and get itching and inflammation when I eat them, but maybe strawberries are your favorite food, and you get so much energy and satisfaction from them.

Learn about your body and build your realistic, most *you* lifestyle.

You Are Not Alone

If you are feeling lost, angry, sad, or hungry—and flipping frustrated with dieting—you are not alone. The weight-loss industry is a multibillion-dollar industry worldwide.

Every year or so, there is a new invention, supplement, hack, or really, really expensive meal plan that guarantees "quick weight loss." (Don't worry, I was scammed too.)

Advertisers and health companies prey on human emotions and the desire to fit the beauty ideal of "thinness" portrayed in the media. However, one of the strongest predictors of weight gain is dieting itself. This fact is swept under the rug as the next new diet appears in the shop window. Who would pay (and not a small amount, might I add) for a new diet if the label read "will help you lose weight the first three months, until the scale triples once you cannot suppress your hunger any longer"?

In reality, food restriction for weight loss is not effective long term, and it causes more harm than good. Take my story, for example: restricting calories led me to bingeing, which introduced me to the world of hunger pains, acne, and worsened periods. Keto led me to overdo the carbs during my binge sprees, which caused me to gain more weight.

The shake diet left me feeling so hungry and unsatisfied with my meals that I would seek satisfaction in my other meals, causing me to overeat and, again, worsen my acne until my face was red all over and painful.

It was only when I began to listen to my body and how I felt after certain meals that I adjusted and tuned into what it was telling me. Because I naturally produce too much estrogen in my body, eating animal protein and dairy with every meal was too heavy for my system and fueled my hormonal issues. Switching to plant-based and dairy-free sources ignited my energy, and my face returned to its normal clear color.

Now, I am not saying that you have to become vegetarian or avoid any specific food group in this book. By no means. If you feel great drinking a glass of milk after dinner, go for it. If you like your weekly steak, dig in. I want you to get back in touch with your body and feel what foods make you feel good, energized, light, and satisfied.

As I mentioned before, there is a term called bio-individuality, which I learned about while getting certified at the Institute for Integrative Nutrition. It means that every single person has unique needs, and those needs change over the course of a lifetime. That is why I like to look at every person's holistic lifestyle to address their concerns and make tailor-made recommendations.

* * *

Claudia, an Olympic gymnast candidate, suffered from issues similar to mine. She was constantly scrutinized by her coaches to lose weight before competitions. Without any professional help, she took to the latest diet craze at the time and went on a shake diet.

It worked for one competition where she lost a total of six pounds as she was able to sustain her hunger pains for two months leading up to it. After the competition, she reported feeling ravenous with hunger and overeating "forbidden foods."

She gained back half the weight she lost in one week and began bingeing on the nights she arrived home from training, her body tired and mind weak from hunger. She overall gained more weight than she lost and felt helpless as the new competition season approached.

Susan, a working mom, always felt unsatisfied with her weight. She believed that if she lost 10 pounds, she would feel better about herself and happy with her appearance.

Susan took to using detox teas to force additional bowel movements. An initial small weight reduction happened, but she noticed after drinking the teas that she constantly had pain in her stomach.

Slowly, over time, she reduced her drinking of the detox teas, but she started struggling to have normal bowel movements again (more on this in the "Difficult Diets" section in the next chapter).

If you feel that your diet is making you feel unworthy of eating, or you feel guilt and shame for eating certain foods … if you are withdrawing socially (avoiding gatherings where food is involved to save calories) … if you have low energy and potentially are using caffeine to stay awake … and/or your metabolism is slowing down … honey, let me tell you, that diet is not for you, as it wasn't for me, Claudia, Susan, and many more like us.

*   *   *

Your body is a fine-tuned working machine. It knows what it needs to run efficiently and optimally. You have just fallen out of rhythm with those signals. There are different systems intertwined in your body—from your blood sugar levels to your hormone signals to your gut microbiome—managed by the big bad boss, your brain.

When something gets off-kilter, the rest of the system tries to compensate, and you enter "survival mode," where your cortisol levels jump off the roof. Not only is this not healthy for your digestion (and can cause long-term GI issues like IBS), but it is not a state your body is designed to live in for long periods of time.

Once you return to normal eating patterns (which will take time, so be patient), you will get back in touch with your body and what it really needs. I am sure you will see the positive effects that take place in your personal, social, and working life the same way I and many of my clients have.

Proper nutrition is so important. It is my mission to educate you on your body and provide tips to get your bodily systems in order so that you can eat without guilt and feel beautiful, energized, and satisfied. So, gorgeous, are you ready to do just that?

NOTE

If you have any medical conditions, please consult with a nutritionally-informed doctor or registered dietitian/health coach to determine the best practices for you and your body. This book contains useful information, facts, and experiences; however, everyone's body is different, and working with a professional can greatly help and answer any lingering questions.

CHAPTER 1

THE REAL REASON DIETING DOESN'T WORK

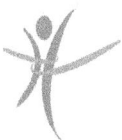

> *"It spills itself in fearing to be spilt."*
> —William Shakespeare

Sarah, a CEO at a large fashion company, would wake up and rush to the office. On her way, she would stop at her nearby Starbucks and get a vanilla latte and blueberry muffin.

For her first meeting, she would have heaps of energy. About an hour later, she would feel a large dip in her energy levels. She would then make her second cup of coffee and go about her usual morning of returning and sending emails.

When lunch came around, she was ravenous. She would eat her chicken pesto pasta with a can of Coke, and she always felt she needed a small chocolate bar to finish off any meal.

Again, she would feel energized for a short period of time until she felt as though she needed a nap. In this scenario, Sarah is experiencing large glucose spikes, explaining the frequent dips in her energy.

Sarah and I have both struggled with our blood sugar levels but in different ways. We'll talk more in the next chapter about how to reduce your glucose spikes so you can get off the energy roller coaster, but before we dive that deep, there's something important we need to address.

Processed foods. If you find yourself craving stuff that makes you feel tired, bloated, or irritable shortly after you've indulged, you need to know that it's not your fault.

Risks of Processed Foods

O' Chips Ahoy, why can't I stop at just one? O'Pringles can, these are too small for just one man. O' Snickers bar, you should come in a big jar … Anyway, I'm not a songwriter, but you get my gist.

Processed foods are addictive. They are designed to be this way in order to get you to buy more (duh). They are usually extremely high in unhealthy forms of salt, sugar, and fat, and they are created using modified ingredients that are easily digestible and taste really good.

The downside to this finger-licking good "food" is that the body has trouble using it, and it gets turned into fat in the liver. It is an unfortunate, sad reality that these are priced lower in comparison to healthier, whole-food alternatives, which is why lower-income earners often turn to processed foods to feed themselves and their families.

Although **sugar** will be discussed in detail in the next chapter, it is worth mentioning here that sugar is one of the most heavily added substances to processed foods. It is also disguised under many different complex names that still sweeten foods and act the same in our bodies. Complicated names like dextrose, lactose, galactose, and maltose are examples and are still, in essence, sugar. (We're onto you, food companies).

Added sugar has no nutritional value and adds to subcutaneous fat (fat around the belly area). The recommended daily allowance is 6 to 9 sugar cubes; it is fair to say that many of the processed food items you find in the grocery store far exceed this in one serving.

Sugar affects the feel-good center in the brain. That's why we associate eating sugary foods with happiness. Consuming them releases dopamine. To continue getting that happiness hit, though, people will add those Oreos, candies, and chocolate bars to their carts in hopes of regaining that oh-so-good feeling.

Oftentimes, when I work with clients, the addiction to sugar can simply be because they are looking for a happiness hit. Working together, we often look at their life on its entire spectrum to determine whether overeating practices may stem from suffering emotional health rather than the body's need for fuel.

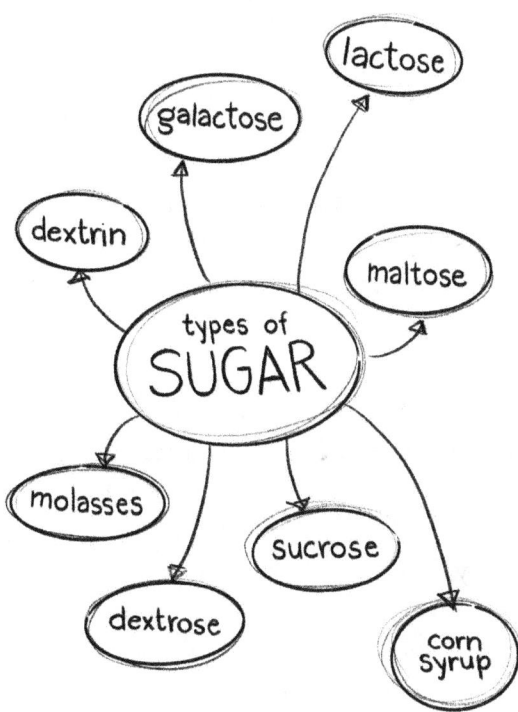

There are other culprits in the food processing industry, and salt is one of them. It does get a bad rap sometimes due to how it shows up obsessively in some items, but it's not all bad.

Salt is needed in our bodies for fluid regulation and nerve impulse transmission; however, too much of it leads to high blood pressure and bloating. This then further ripples out to arterial damage that restricts oxygen and forces the heart to work harder.

The recommended daily allowance is about 2300 mg per day, but again, to hell with numbers. Once you fall back in tune with your body, you will be able to feel when you might be eating too much salt or sugar because it will affect how you feel and perform (more on this in the energetics section).

In essence, processed foods create a vicious cycle of a momentary feel-good sensation, followed by feelings of heaviness and sluggishness from the low energetics these foods hold. To regain those positive feelings, more processed food is bought and ingested, and these processed food companies are sitting pretty.

Getting back to whole foods is the ultimate goal. I know it doesn't sound exciting, but give it a try. In the beginning, it might feel bland after your taste buds have become used to that sugar or salt hit, but over time, they will become more sensitive, and you will love the feeling and high energy levels you have.

NOTE

I am not telling you to never pick up a chocolate bar again or to put down that can of Pringles. By no means, I am not a monster. I enjoy treats when my body craves them. The difference is that it is not a staple in my diet, nor an everyday encounter. Instead, I now make any baked goods I am craving as I can control the amount of sugar inside (which you can receive in the recipes I incorporate into my programs as a resource to my clients, as well as an abundance of other tools)! Although I love that brief happiness hit, I know that I will feel a bit bloated and sluggish afterward. And that's ok … sometimes. Grab my recipes at the link below!

http://thisisntadiet.com/apps/recipe/

Difficult Diets

Let's talk about the D word. **Diets**. As you read from my story, I have a particular problem with this word and way of thinking. It has caused me and many others like me unnecessary headaches, shame, embarrassment, guilt, and weight gain.

Diets are concerned with short-term weight loss; they are not sustainable, and they only deal with one side of the equation and not the whole formula.

There is a theory called the **set point theory**. It states that we each have a genetically determined range of weight that our bodies are programmed to protect. This point is reflected in genetics, diet changes, activity, lifestyle, the environment, and stress levels.

Once the brain detects that fat levels have fallen below the established level, it adjusts certain hormones to burn energy more slowly and increase calorie intake.

(**Note:** This theory is regarding a survival mechanism your body has from ancient times when food was scarce. And let's just say that food isn't so scarce nowadays.)

This theory makes sense in practice. Many dieters enter starvation mode, and then their bodies tell them to overeat to counteract and protect their set point. This is not to say that you cannot improve your body, but it is a theory that diets don't want you to know about, as it sets people on the path toward body acceptance.

You should also know that your weight can fluctuate from 2 to 6 pounds every day depending on various factors, which is why the scale is not a realistic indicator of what is going on with your body.

Let's take an in-depth look at some of the diets you might have encountered before or might currently be on.

Calorie Counting

Calorie counting is a solid fallback option for most dieters. This method places less emphasis on food quality and more on a numerical basis for weighing foods against one another.

A classic example is that two slices of chocolate can equate to the same number of calories as the average-sized banana. One is packed full of sugar, dairy, and additives and will do nothing for my appetite, whereas the other is enriched with potassium, healing benefits, and fiber to keep me full for longer.

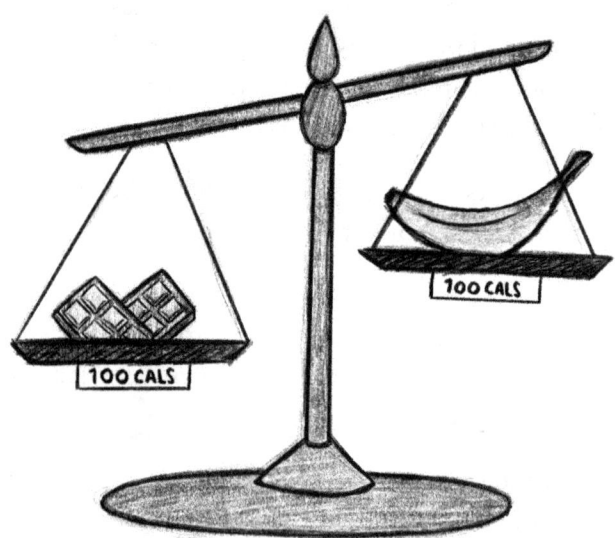

Although calorie counting, in theory, makes sense, it emphasizes the wrong aspects of nutrition, and it also causes feelings of guilt for those who are trying to stick to their daily allotted calories but are still hungry with no calories left, raiding the pantry for chocolate to shadow their guilt.

If your body is still hungry, it probably has a good reason, such as needing more fuel. Allowing yourself to eat when your body is cuing you will remove the gleam and shine of unhealthy options. Sure, if you want them, go ahead. But without food restrictions, healthier options tend to become closer friends.

Liquid Diets

Here come the **liquid diets**—those short-term weight loss, binge-eating guarantees. There is a natural loss of nutrients in this chosen diet, as chewing helps with nutrient absorption. Fiber, the key to feeling full, is also lost when fiber-rich foods are blended or juiced.

When I did my shake diet, I would have my lunchtime shake followed by bread and chocolate to curb my hunger pains (it sounds a bit counterproductive, but to me at the time, it seemed like a good idea).

Needless to say, I was a bit heavier coming off this plan, as well as other athletes like our Olympic gymnast example, Claudia. It is also important to note that many shake powders contain artificial ingredients and added sugars to enhance their taste (again coming back to our processed food discussion).

Keto Diet

Now we come to one of my favorites. This one has tricked millions worldwide into eating all of the fatty foods they desire, just the kick is that they can't have any carbs. You know who I'm talking about. Let me introduce **Keto**!

(As I write this, I almost feel sick thinking of some keto recipes I have seen online—cheese steak wrapped up with bacon and dipped in mayonnaise—yuck.)

Keto is a low-carb diet designed to burn fat for energy. However, people often report having low energy levels and increased cravings. A Harvard medical study concluded that due to Keto's restrictive nature, 50% of the people were unable to follow the diet past six months.

There are also reported statistics of a higher cholesterol and salt intake. (No kidding, imagine eating that recipe above every day.) One reason why people on keto lose weight quickly is due to the rapid loss in water weight caused by the reduced intake of carbs (which isn't really weight loss; you're gonna gain that back quickly). In the same Harvard study, the Keto diet market was valued at $10.22 billion in 2019 and was expected to grow 5.3% annually. Talk about fooling a whole lot of people.

Neuropeptide Y is the chemical produced in the brain that triggers our drive to eat carbs. When we underfeed that drive, this chemical empowers the body to seek out higher amounts of carbohydrates, leading to the eventual dilemma of overeating.

It is important for me to say that carbs are not the enemy. I used to think this way. There was a four-year period when I did not touch bread, pasta, or rice. However, now I eat pasta at least twice a week, bread almost every day, and rice as an occasional side.

Carbohydrates are fuel for your body, and in the next chapter, I will help you with tricks to eat your carbs and curb your glucose spikes. Keto is also associated with the risk of getting kidney stones, osteoporosis, hyperlipidemia, and impaired growth.

It also decreases athletic/exercise performance in both men and women, and it deprives the body of many key nutrients like potassium, thiamin, folate, vitamins A, E, and B6, and calcium due to the lack of vegetables and fruits present in the diet.

Mike, one of my old friends, was a university student at the time and was trying to lose his wintertime bulk by dropping a couple of pounds for summer. He started implementing the Keto diet into his lifestyle.

The first few weeks, he felt irritable and angry as his body craved carbs for energy, but Mike resisted. During exam season he could barely focus on studying and had to drink energy drinks to focus. He began to drop several pounds within his second and third weeks as his body entered a state of ketosis (where your body is using fats for fuel instead of glucose).

Mike was finally happy with his body and decided to go back to his original diet as he missed his usual bread, pasta, and pizza, which he would eat some nights of the week. Mike gained back the weight he lost two-fold as he overate carbohydrates because of his large cravings.

Keto is even more damaging for women as it can mess with our delicate hormonal balance.

Detox Diets

Detox diets are another fad dieting trend. They are usually sold with teas that provide short-term weight loss as they are laced with laxatives like senna, an ingredient that irritates the stomach lining to stimulate a bowel movement, causing dehydration, cramps, diarrhea, and the depletion of key minerals.

Laxatives are dangerous as excessive use can stop your bowels from functioning normally. Not to mention, your body already has a natural detox process. Your liver naturally changes toxins to less harmful substances to be excreted via stool or skin sweat; therefore, while you may see short-term weight loss with these plans, they can actually be incredibly detrimental to your health and cause implications down the road.

Natural detox methods can be extremely beneficial, such as properly washing fruits and vegetables to get rid of pesticides, using an air and water filter to avoid heavy metal toxins, going for sauna sessions a couple of times per week, and supporting your liver in its detox process by waking up and drinking a glass of warm water and lemon.

There is one thought on eating that I hold true to my heart because it has worked for me. I do not support you going vegetarian simply because of my success story. I merely mean to highlight the benefits of the lifestyle, as there are many, and perhaps turn you on to some plant-based protein options occasionally. (However, if you are a die-hard meat eater, you have my full support, as everyone's body is different and may require different nutrition plans.)

Plant-Based

One of the reasons I chose a primarily plant-based way of eating is that going plant-based reduces the environmental impact. There are huge amounts of water that go into the animal protein sector, not to mention all the hormones added by humans and genetically modified crops to feed animals and fatten them up, which throws off the entire ecosystem.

If you, a potential regular meat-eater, went one day of your week without meat, you would feed 100 million other people on the planet who do not have access to certain resources (money or enough water or grain to feed livestock). You would also save deforestation in the Amazon as many parts of that rainforest are cut down and burned to create vegetation where cattle livestock are then introduced to keep up with the growing demand for meat worldwide. But hey, don't take my word for it. Check out this insightful documentary on Netflix called *You Are What You Eat: A Twin Experiment*.

Plant-based items typically cost less, and there are healthier weights reported on these diets, as well as lower risks of diabetes, cardiovascular diseases, and cancers.

The documentary also showed how grocery stores are legally allowed to accept poultry products that have 25% pathogens. One out of every 25 chickens bought in grocery stores has salmonella[1], and one out of five

---

[1] Salmonella: a bacteria in the gut that causes food poisoning.

has E.Coli[2] due to the horrible living conditions in which these livestock are bred.

A CAFO chicken farm (meaning that it has over 1,000 chickens) will put 30,000 chickens into one barn that has 20,000 sq ft. Every chicken has 0.67 square feet of space, and they, therefore, run around in their feces and climb all over each other, causing open wounds leading to infection. If you do eat chicken, at least get it from a local organic or biodynamic farm that promotes humane conditions.

Stay away from farmed salmon, though. Just imagine dozens of nets with thousands of fish that are bred, overnourished, and that swim around in their feces. Usually, when they are fished, they have large sores over their body and are much fatter than wild-caught salmon (proven to hold more fat than a McDonald's cheeseburger, crazy). Always look for wild-caught fish when buying fish at the grocery store.

This is the scary reality we live in, and it is one major reason why I went vegetarian. You truly can't trust that what you buy in grocery stores is safe. Going vegetarian has worked for me, but it might not work for you.

I have included many tricks and hacks in this book that do not pertain to being a vegetarian that you can use to help you on your health journey. These strategies will be outlined at the end to support all your different bodily systems.

But before we get into the health hacks, let's go back to the basics for a minute.

The Basics

There is a lot of information available today regarding calories, macros, and your overall digestion process, but the reality is that most of it that

---

[2] E.Coli: bacteria found in the intestines of humans and other animals which in severe cases can cause food poisoning.

is known in today's society is off the packaging of a shiny new meal plan. Needless to say, some of it may be falsified or exaggerated to sell the next "miracle" weight-loss program. Yawn.

Calories

Calories are units of energy. It takes calories to breathe, circulate blood, process nutrients, and create cells. You are probably familiar with the calories on the nutrition label of a food item or through constantly counting your daily calories (probably trying to squeeze into that dangerous 1,200 calorie range, which is leading you into starvation mode and, no doubt, binges).

Calories are regarded in the dieting world as the savior of weight loss. "You can eat whatever you want, as long as it fits within your daily calorie limitation" … This is so painfully wrong, as we will explore in later chapters, that it is not just the quantity of what you are eating that is important for you and your health, but the quality.

For example, artificial sweeteners have zero calories, however, they change metabolic pathways in gut microbes so that they produce more short-chain fatty acids which are absorbed by the colon, adding additional calories. In short, what is categorized as zero calories on a package, in reality contains some through natural bodily reactions. A little lesson to not trust everything you read on packaging labels.

Science has proven that certain foods feed your fat cells more than others (mostly those processed packaged foods we have brought into our diet as a staple). For example, if I eat a 100-calorie chocolate bar (which is full of many additives and ingredients I can't even pronounce) every day instead of a 100-calorie banana (which contains fiber, protein, vitamins, and minerals), over time, I would gain body fat, even though I ate the same number of calories.

Did I just shock one of your core beliefs about nutrition and food? I flipping hope so!

Macros (Carbohydrates, Protein, and Fat)

You are probably also familiar with the three macros (maybe you also count them): carbohydrates, protein, and fat. Carbohydrates hold four calories per gram, proteins four calories per gram, and fats come in at a whopping nine calories per gram. And no, you should not avoid fats just because they have more calories; they are important for your health too.

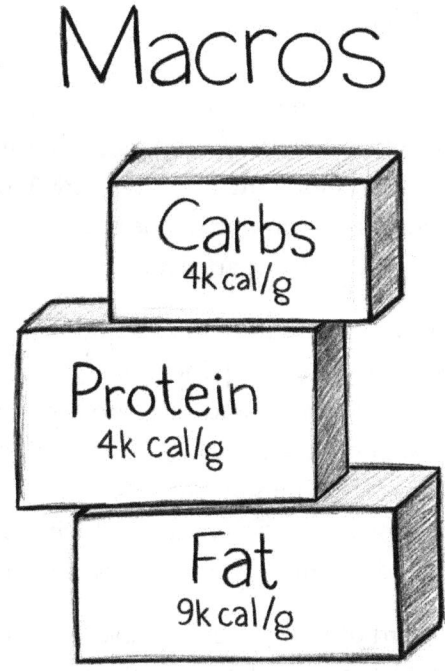

Carbohydrates are our main energy source. They also help regulate brain function and provide us with the happy hormone serotonin, which is released when we eat them.

The carbohydrate digestion process starts with them being broken down into simple carbs, and all non-glucose monosaccharides[3] are converted into glucose in the liver, which is released into the bloodstream. This

---

[3] Monosaccharide: the simplest form of sugar which forms the basis of any carbohydrate.

glucose can either be used immediately if the body is active, or stored in the liver and muscles as glycogen (more on this in the next chapter).

It is important to note that fiber is also a carb, however, the digestion process differs. You'll learn more on all things blood-sugar related in the next chapter—not giving anything away yet!

Proteins are the building blocks of our cells, forming the structure of tissues, carrying molecules where they are needed, and producing and deploying hormones. It's important to note and get around the stigma that protein solely comes from animal tissues. On the contrary, animals obtain their proteins from plants. Many of the strongest animals are herbivores (sorry for the short but important PSA on plant protein). Gorillas, elephants, and rhinoceros are all herbivores, and I'd say they are not doing too badly in the size department.

Plants synthesize proteins and amino acids and can be found in many leafy green sources, beans, lentils, quinoa, nuts, and seeds, and the list goes on and on. On the other hand, fats are a macro that promotes weight balance and support for the cardiovascular system, and they are needed to absorb fat-soluble vitamins such as A, D, E, and K. Fats, when digested, are broken down into triglycerides, which are a type of glucose. They travel in the bloodstream to where they will be used and stored.

You have probably heard of trans, saturated, and unsaturated fats, but you may be wondering which are good and which are sinful according to the latest TikTok influencer. It can be confusing to make sense of all the information out there when one day one thing is the latest health craze, and the next there are studies coming out as to why it will actually harm your health.

Here is what I know to be true:

Trans fats are also called PHOs or partially hydrogenated oils because they started out as oil but, after being hydrogenated, changed into a solid fat at room temperature. They can be found usually in processed foods to increase the shelf life. Most fast food is fried in trans fat. Because it can elevate bad cholesterol, raising the chance of cardiovascular diseases, it's best to avoid this type of fat. Read labels and choose brands without partially hydrogenated oil.

Saturated fats are also solid at room temperature; however, there is mixed evidence as to whether it is coined a healthy or unhealthy fat. What's clear is that a diet high in saturated fats from fried foods, sugary baked goods, and fast food is unhealthy, whereas natural saturated fats from a diet of grass-fed dairy and meat, nuts, and coconut are healthy options.

Unsaturated fats are liquid at room temperature. They lower bad cholesterol and improve the control of blood sugar. The two types that exist are **monounsaturated fats** and **polyunsaturated fats**, and they are generally found in foods like avocados, olives, peanut butter, fatty fish, and nuts and seeds.

Now that we have covered our macro bases, I think it's time we address the elephant in the room: cholesterol—the dreaded and fearful cholesterol. Most of us know it is harmful to our bodies, especially to our cardiovascular systems. Would it surprise you if I told you that there is also a good form of cholesterol? (I know, right, shocking).

Cholesterol

Cholesterol[4] is used in the body to help build cells, and there are two types. The first is HDL[5], which is the good form of cholesterol. It positively affects the body as it holds more protein, is anti-inflammatory, and carries LDL[6] cholesterol (bad cholesterol) away from arteries to the liver.

LDL is the second type, and it negatively affects the body as it sticks to the inside walls of arteries and causes a buildup of fatty material, thereby limiting blood flow.

---

[4] Cholesterol: substance made by your liver that is found in all cells of your body.
[5] HDL cholesterol: high-density lipoprotein. This good cholesterol removes cholesterol from the body back to the liver where it can be removed from your system.
[6] LDL cholesterol: low-density lipoprotein—too much LDL cholesterol can cause a buildup in arteries and can lead to coronary diseases.

Trans fats and potentially some saturated fat sources can increase levels of LDL and decrease levels of HDL, which is why processed foods hold a dangerous underlying tone (more on this in the next section of this chapter) and why food quality is not addressed enough in today's nutrition.

Vitamins

Two types of vitamins exist: water-soluble and fat-soluble. Water-soluble vitamins are those that are lost through fluids and must be replenished every day. These are vitamins like the various B vitamins as well as vitamin C.

This is why, for athletes and dancers, a good vitamin complex filled with water-soluble vitamins is key to maintaining performance and daily bodily functions due to the high volume loss of fluids daily.

Fat-soluble vitamins accumulate in the body and are not needed every day. These are vitamins like vitamins A, E, D, and K.

Minerals

When it comes to minerals, there are a lot of mix-ups in the thinking between vitamins and minerals. I often hear, "Well, they're the same thing, aren't they?" No, minerals are organic compounds. They are made by plants, soil, rock, or water. Minerals are essential for cell processes, fluid balance, nervous system function, and bone structure.

You have definitely heard of minerals before when self-diagnosing over Google that you may have low iron levels or that all of the fitness icons are taking magnesium supplements, so you should too. Again, everybody's bodies are different.

While it may not be harmful to take a vitamin or mineral supplement, it is best to obtain your nutrients from food and to do so, increase the variety of color on your plate. This is a surefire way to obtain different vitamins and minerals without downing nine different pills every morning and spending a hefty sum of money on supplements you might not even need—especially if you already eat a balanced diet.

Hydration

Last but not least, hydration—the Hail Mary of nutrition. No, but really, all sarcasm aside, staying hydrated is in your best interest. Hydration enables the circulatory system to carry essential oxygen and nutrients to cells. It also filters out waste products from kidneys and regulates mood, concentration, productivity, and appetite.

A little fun fact is that your brain's hunger and thirst signals are the same. Many times, when you feel hungry, you are confusing your bodily cues with those of thirst. The next time you want to grab a snack and you feel you might be out of sync with your body messages, try this trick.

Imagine it's 2 p.m., and you had lunch two hours ago. You are feeling a bit peckish for a little snacky snack. First, stop that hand from reaching for that sweet treat (more on this in the next chapter), and instead, grab a glass of water and wait 20 minutes.

There is a time lapse between your body's signals and realizations, so if after the 20 minutes pass, you still feel hungry, go ahead and grab that snacky snack. But, if it has subsided, you will realize your body was simply just crying out for some water.

As you continue to learn more about your body and its functions and you continue to go about your daily life, you will start to notice these cues, and you will be able to implement these little tricks to help you on your way to becoming more alert on what your body is telling you it needs.

Now it's time to get into the fun stuff … tips and tricks for helping your body stay energized without fad diets, restricting calories, or eliminating your favorite foods.

Let's dance, shall we?

CHAPTER 2

GET YOUR GLUCOSE IN CHECK

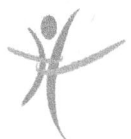

"Slow and steady wins the race."

—Aesop

My friend Karen, a dancer like myself, would always arrive home from training feeling hungry. Her usual go-to was pasta with tomato sauce, which she would prepare before leaving. She would serve herself a large portion and dig in.

She would feel full for just over an hour until her hunger signals returned. She would then serve herself a smaller pasta portion once again and have some chocolate afterward as a sweet treat.

Karen could never understand why she would never feel satisfied for the rest of the night until I suggested she add fiber and protein to her meal and eat them in the correct order.

Making this one change had Karen feeling full without taking her pasta away, might I add, and solved her constant reappearing cravings. Karen also noticed a weight reduction of five pounds after one month through the lessened cravings and added fiber and protein to her meals, which decreased her overall limitless consumption per night.

You see, I am a huge believer in non restriction. Once I learned this tip, it was a game-changer for me! I was like: "You're telling me I can have my cake and eat it too? What's the catch?" The catch is that there isn't one!

As long as you are getting adequate fiber, protein, and fat into your diet, adding a bit of carbs won't cause any harm. That's why whole grain bread, occasional pasta nights, and home-baked pastries are a staple in our household. These are simple joys in my life and now non negotiables for me.

It is crazy to think back to just two or three years ago when I was scared to even add a bit of rice to my plate. The thought of eating a bowl of pasta to me seemed like a sin. I've come so far to heal my relationship with food and educate myself on what a healthy lifestyle and mindset actually look like.

This is the work we do at This Isn't a Diet, and my clients see not only weight loss, but they look at food in a completely new light and develop new and improved mindsets about their health on a full spectrum.

Glucose Symptom Checklist

Glucose is one of the most important topics of this book. That's right, one of the big kahunas. You have probably heard of the term **glucose** before. Perhaps it has been used interchangeably with sugar and thrown about loosely in conversations or articles you may have heard or read.

It is indeed a large topic, and there is often a lot of miscommunication about it. In fact, every second your body burns about eight billion molecules of glucose.

With something that we truly use to its fullest, shouldn't we know more about the subject? Before we dive in too far, I have included a checklist to see if you have some of these symptoms and should take steps to level off your glucose spikes (which are included at the end of this chapter).

Please tick the box if you have this symptom. If you tick more than four boxes, you might suffer from sporadic glucose spikes throughout your day and want to pay close attention to the tips toward the end of this chapter.

Constant hunger ☐

Cravings ☐

Fatigue ☐

Poor sleep ☐

Prone to sickness ☐

Gut issues ☐

Depression ☐

Acne ☐

Chronic inflammation ☐

Arthritis ☐

Stubborn weight ☐

The Four Types of Sugars

There are four types of sugars, and each impacts blood sugar levels differently. First, we have **starch**. Starch turns to glucose in the mouth and gut through the aid of saliva. In more technical terms, alpha-amylase[7] snaps the bonds of the chain and frees glucose molecules.

Secondly, we have **fructose**. When you eat a piece of fruit, you are eating fructose. This consists of unchained glucose molecules, so when you bite

---
[7] Alpha-amylase: enzymes that catabolize and hydrolyze linkages of starch to release glucose.

into that piece of fruit, it immediately tastes sweet. This is why, back in the day, people knew which fruits were safe to eat, as those with poisonous properties tended to have a stronger, bitter taste.

After you eat fructose, the body turns a portion of it back into glucose in the small intestine and does not need insulin to be absorbed to process it (more on this in a moment).

Thirdly, we have **sucrose**. This can be found naturally in certain plant foods, and when ingested, it is broken down into equal parts of glucose and fructose.

Finally, we have **fiber** last, but certainly not least. This important component is special in that during digestion, it does not get turned back into glucose. Instead, it remains intact as fiber until it reaches the colon and excretion.

Fiber is important for slowing down the rate of stomach emptying and reducing glucose absorption. This important sugar is the key to the journey we are going on. It will keep you feeling full longer and, through proper use, will help you eat those sweet treats I know you love.

Types of Sugars	Digestion Process	Is it turned into glucose?
Starch	Turns to glucose in the mouth through saliva. Chained bonds are snapped, and glucose is freed.	Yes
Fructose	Unchained molecules. In the small intestine, it is partially turned back to glucose.	Partially

Sucrose	Broken down into equal parts glucose and fructose in the body.	Partially
Fiber	Digested and remains as fiber until excretion.	No

These descriptions are quite vague and simplified toward the actual bodily processes that go on within us, but they give a general, useful understanding.

It is important to know as well that most starchy parts of plants are processed to make processed foods. Usually, they are stripped of their fiber, and extra sugars are added.

Processed food companies do this because when we eat sugar, dopamine floods the brain. It is the same rush as when we have sex, take drugs, scroll through social media, or drink. And then you want more, and more, and more, and more, until you find yourself bulk buying sugary processed foods multiple times per week. It becomes addictive, which is why these large food companies are so profitable. They prey on our natural bodily processes to create induced cravings.

Glucose Spikes

In her book *Glucose Revolution*, Jessie Inchauspé discusses **glucose spikes**[8] and their drastic effects on the body. It truly revolutionized the topic and research of blood sugar for me, and it was one of the first steps on my road to self-discovery.

In my health journey, I could never understand why I never felt full, why I always had cravings, why I was putting on weight, eating the same things as others, and why I could finish a box of chocolates any day of the week with no problem. I knew deep down that I was

---

[8] Glucose spike: a sharp rise and decline of glucose levels following a meal or snack.

missing some piece of information regarding the topic of glucose, so I started looking.

First, a healthy glucose level is defined by The American Diabetes Association as a 60-100 mg/dL level when you wake up. (If your level is between 100-126 mg/dL, it is a pre-indicator of diabetes.) Unless you wear a glucose monitor, this won't make any sense to you. No worries, girl, let's make it make sense.

As we take in food, our glucose levels will naturally rise and then return to normal or fall based on certain conditions. Think of it like this:

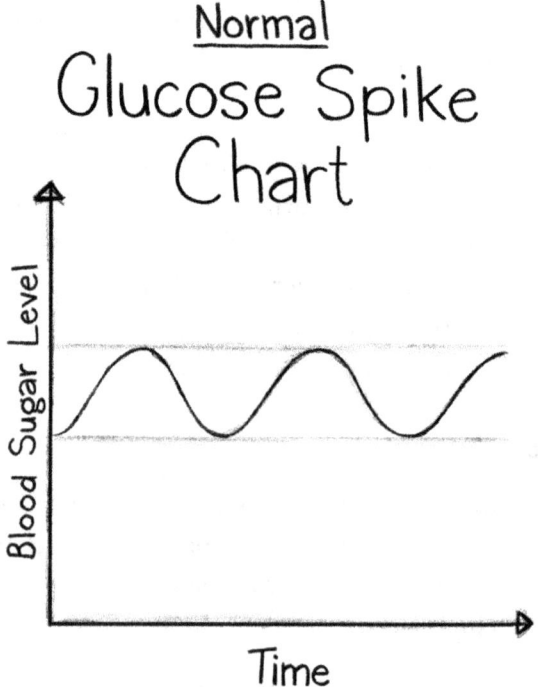

This is a sample glucose chart of an average person and their food intake between waking up and having lunch. This is aimed at depicting the fluctuating levels of glucose that occur in our bodies from hour to hour and between feeding times.

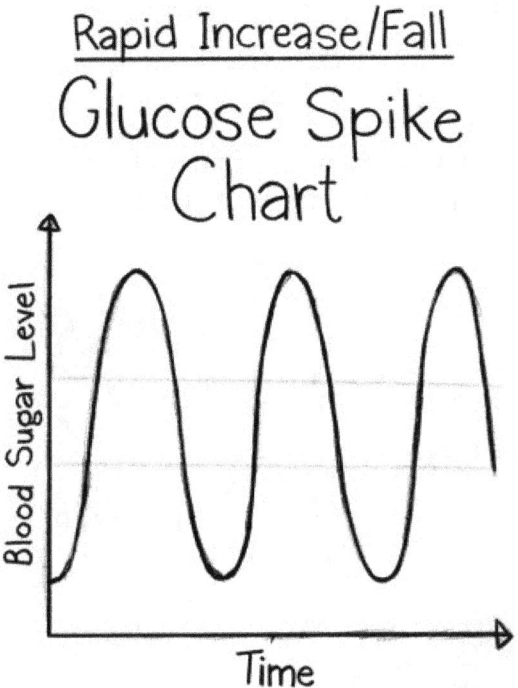

This is an example of Sarah's drastic glucose spike chart after her sugary breakfast and the large drop she experienced afterward.

It is important to note that high fluctuations in glucose spikes, such as Sarah's example, are harmful. Spikes are classified as rapid increases and drops in glucose concentrations after eating. The goal is not to increase glucose levels by 30 mg/dL after eating (again, if that doesn't make sense, that's ok. Basically, our goal is to make this curve as flat as possible).

There will be tools outlined to help achieve this. Before we get further into why glucose spikes are harmful, it is useful to know that there are slow glucose burners and fast glucose burners.

Think of it like this. In a running race, there are slow runners and there are fast runners. The fast runners get in and get out. They do their job efficiently and don't cause any delays.

The slow runners obviously stay on the track for a longer period of time, causing a queue of people waiting to start their next race.

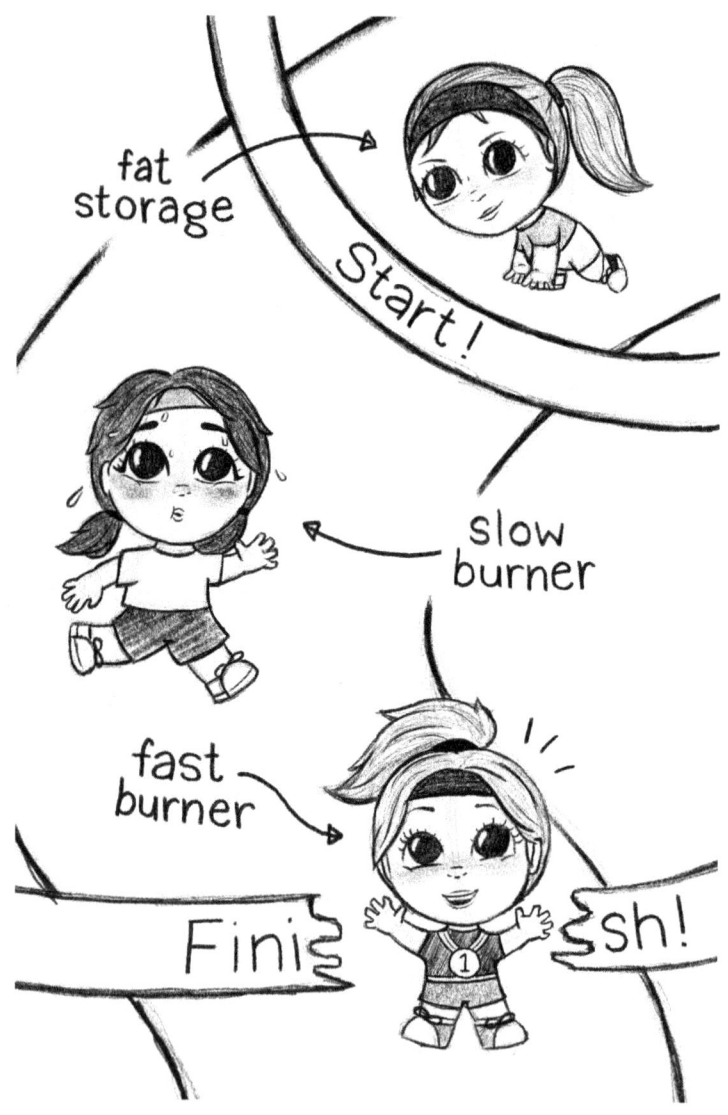

In this scenario, the track is your insulin receptor, and the runners are the little glucose molecules running to do their job. The runners in line for their next race are the glucose molecules waiting to be used. They are currently stored in fat cells, out of the way of the race, and free from damage in the body.

So, to sum up, if you are a slow burner, your system is just a bit delayed in processing glucose. As you continue to eat, a line of glucose molecules will wait for their race but have to wait at their starting line in your fat cells.

Now, for you fast burners out there, just know that I am sooo envious of you, as I myself am a slow burner. Fast burners are those people who lose weight easily.

When I was in my dieting craze and would see people around me eating chocolate and chips and pizza and still losing weight, I honestly couldn't handle it. We all know of someone like this, and we all secretly wish deep down that one day, their eating choices will catch up to them.

However, being a fast burner also comes with some difficulties. Fast burners usually feel anxious or dizzy when hypoglycemic, and they overheat with little exertion.

I'm sure by now, you can get a sense of which category you fall into. It usually derives from generations of ancestral eating patterns and how your genetics have formed you. With the upcoming tools in one of the next sections, we will cover several tips to help, but first, we should get back into the glucose spike explanation.

Do you remember from science class that one piece of useless information about the mitochondria? Well, we are about to use that piece of information. As glucose is ingested and begins to flood cells, it heads to the mitochondria[9] to power daily processes. However, the mitochondria

---

[9] Mitochondria: cell organelles that generate chemical energy to power cells.

can only burn as much glucose as the cell needs for energy, not more, not less.

When we encounter a glucose spike, glucose floods the cells too quickly, leaving the mitochondria with too much unnecessary glucose (like having too many runners wanting to run the same race on a small track).

This then releases free radicals[10] as a result, and fat becomes stored in fat cells. Free radicals are dangerous for the body. They harm anything they touch, especially our genetic code. When free radicals harm our genetic code, they can cause mutations, aiding in the development of cancer.

Oxidative stress[11] will then set in. This becomes the main driver of heart disease, type 2 diabetes, cognitive decline, and, yes, ladies, aging. We refer to this process as glycation, the unavoidable browning process that happens inside of us that can be sped up or slowed down.

As glucose and fructose molecules bump into other molecules, they become glycated, leading to increased browning (perhaps like when there are too many runners who might step on and injure each other during the race … I'm doing the best I can, guys, with this example).

Other lifestyle choices, such as smoking and exposure to UV rays, will also increase the rate of glycation. Once a molecule is glycated, it is damaged forever (like a lifelong running injury—after an irreversible break or tear, that person is not going to be able to run again, and they might even have difficulty walking).

That's the power your lifestyle choices have over the health of your insides. And a key piece of the puzzle is that fructose molecules glycate things 10x as fast as glucose. This is crazy to even think about, as many

---

[10] Free radical: atom or molecule that contains one or more unpaired electrons and can exist independently.
[11] Oxidative stress: an imbalance between free radicals and antioxidants in the body.

of the additives found in processed foods nowadays are fructose (given that it tastes sweet instantly). Hopefully, this will make you think twice when you go grocery shopping.

Now, as with everything, there are short-term and long-term effects. You might relate to several of these effects and be able to use the tools outlined in this book to remedy them:

Short-Term Effects of Glucose Spikes	Long-Term Effects of Glucose Spikes
Constant Hunger	Acne
Many cravings	Aging and arthritis
Chronic fatigue (like Sarah, too much glucose means energy production is compromised).	Chronic inflammation and oxidative stress on the brain (this can lead to Alzheimer's and dementia, which can become reversible when glucose levels are evened out).
Poor sleep	Cancer risk
Chronic colds and illnesses (with many glucose spikes, our immune system becomes faulty).	Depression
Worsened menopause	Gut issues
Impaired memory and cognitive function	Infertility and polycystic ovarian syndrome (insulin and sex organs decide whether the body is a safe place to conceive).

Insulin

In walks our handy sidekick, Mr. **Insulin**, an essential little helper. His job is to stash excess glucose and tuck it away into storage units. This occurs when glucose levels increase, and this hormone is secreted by the pancreas. Glucose is stored in storage units to keep it out of circulation and to protect it from damage.

Insulin is equivalent to springtime. We all know too well the relief of the warm weather and packing boxes of our winter clothes to tuck them away until next year. Your body does the same. It packs those tight little boxes, organizes them, and shelves them for later. Now, where is this glucose stored, might you ask? Well, now it will make sense why too much sugar can lead to weight gain.

Glucose is stored in the liver and muscles, and when those are at capacity, it's stored in fat cells. Fructose, however, is special. Fructose can only be stored as fat. Once too much fat accumulates in the liver, it may lead to the development of nonalcoholic fatty liver disease.

Glucose stored in the liver is turned into a type of starch called glycogen, which, once transformed, does no damage. Because insulin is sent out when glucose levels are too high, this causes insulin spikes that coincide with glucose spikes. It is, therefore, desirable to try to get a flatter glucose curve, which will naturally flatten insulin curves.

Think of it like storing your winter clothes. All your coats and sweaters take up space, so it's easy to fill an entire closet. If you don't have enough space for them, you'll end up with winter clothes boxes all over the house. Imagine finding piles of clothes in your kitchen and bathroom (a.k.a. in your fat stores, where nobody wants them or needs them).

Maybe you are having an "aha" moment, or maybe you knew this already. Either way, it's incredibly useful information for making more educated choices.

If weight/fat loss is your goal, you should instead focus on lowering your insulin levels, as your "fat-burning" mode activates when your insulin is low. In this mode, glycogen is retransformed back into glucose and used up until fat stores are tapped into.

From our spring cleaning example, think of it like giving some of your winter clothes to charity. You have less stuff laying around your house, and it's much easier to manage! I know this might sound like keto, but believe me, it is not. You can achieve this while still eating carbohydrates and sugar; just follow the tips in the next section.

5 Key Tips to Minimize Glucose Curves

Inchauspé details 10 tips in her glucose book to minimize the spike of glucose (and therefore insulin) curves. These tips do not take away or restrict food groups, and it is clear and achievable. I will share with you five of the tips I, and many of my clients, have found to be the most beneficial, from our own experiences.

Hack 1: Eat Foods in the Right Order

As we discussed in the beginning, there are four different types of sugars, fiber being one of the most beneficial of them all.

Inchauspé detailed that if what's on your plate is eaten in a certain order, you can reduce your overall glucose spike by 73% and your insulin curve by 48%. Those are not bad numbers. And, best of all, you don't have to restrict or change anything that is on your plate.

Sounds better than that latest dieting plan, no? The right order for eating consists of fiber first, protein and fats second, and starches and sugars last. Now, why does this work?

If carbs are eaten first, they will cause a sharp spike immediately as there is nothing yet in the stomach to slow down the effects of glucose and because glucose sensitivity is higher (especially in the mornings when you are in a fasted state).

Eating fiber first permits a solid layer in your stomach and bloodstream, which you can then begin to layer with other foods and your eventual sugars. Think of leafy greens and cruciferous vegetables. These are perfect to start your meal.

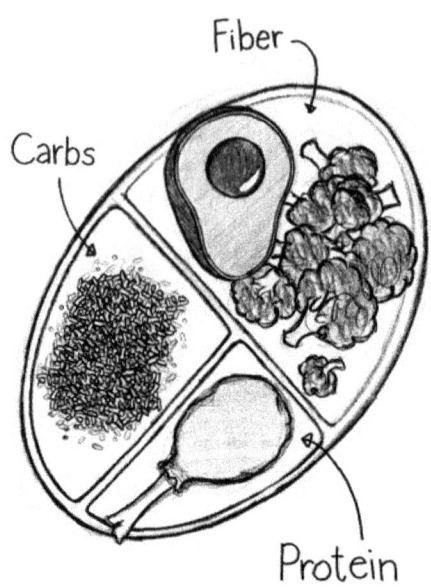

This is a clear plate example containing fiber, protein, fats, and carbs. The broccoli, which contains fiber, should be eaten first, followed by the chicken (protein) and the avocado (healthy fats), succeeded by carbohydrates (the rice-quinoa blend).

Fiber reduces the action of alpha-amylase, which essentially helps break down starches (remember the first type of sugar we talked about) into sugar's simplest form, glucose.

We want this to be reduced and slowed down so that glucose doesn't enter and overwhelm your system too quickly and so food can stay in your tummy longer. When your mom told you to eat your veggies, she was onto something.

Let's take a food example to demonstrate this. Let's say your lunch was chicken pasta with broccoli. If you deconstruct that meal, you have your fiber, your protein, and your carbs.

First, you should start with the broccoli to build a layer of fiber in your stomach. Next, eat the chicken. The last thing should be the pasta; once there is enough of a base in your tummy as it makes it more difficult for glucose to enter the bloodstream.

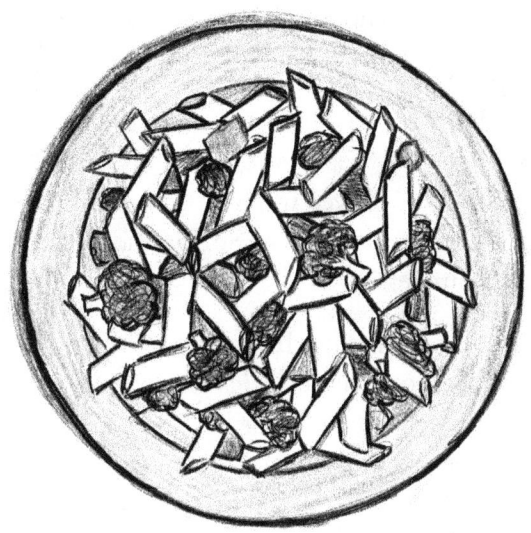

This is a depiction of chicken and broccoli pasta. If you were to start with the pasta in this picture, it would ignite cravings soon after, as eating starches and sugars first returns the hunger hormone ghrelin in two hours.

Now, you might see from this picture that everything is mixed. What should you do in this scenario? Well, you should strive to combine your starches, sugars, fats, and proteins and not eat "naked" carbs.

Therefore, eating the broccoli and pasta together will have a counteracting effect. Eating carbs alone causes sharp spikes; however, when eaten with something else, it limits the altitude of the spike to avoid spike charts like Sarah's.

Hack 2: Flatten Your Breakfast Curve

When we wake up, our bodies are what we call in a fasted state. This makes it more sensitive to whatever you first decide to eat. (It is true what they say, "breakfast is the most important meal of the day.")

Many people nowadays are in a rush in the mornings. They look for something quick that they can either pick up on the way (ex., a coffee and a sugary muffin) or simply pour themselves a quick bowl of cereal. Both examples have high sugar content and do not fit the first hack of food order.

If these types of sugary carbohydrates are eaten first thing in the morning, you set yourself up for constant hunger and cravings for the rest of the day. That's why savory breakfast options are best. Choosing savory over sweet flattens glucose curves and has been proven to increase cognitive performance throughout the day. So, instead of that bowl of cereal, perhaps prepare an omelet.

I was a classic example of making this mistake. When I was in my beginner dieter phase, I was counting calories and basically trying to eat less. Now, I am one of those rare morning birds you hear so much about. I love to wake up before everyone else, make myself breakfast, and take my time in the morning. (It's one of my favorite pleasures.)

I used to try to eat a lot in the morning so I could skip lunch and save calories. Usually, I would start my day off with a *big* bowl of oatmeal. This oatmeal was topped with different fruits and lots, and lots, and lots of honey. It was one of my favorite breakfasts (and I still eat it from time to time using my fourth hack, which will come soon), but my master plan didn't work.

Not only was I ravenous for lunch, but I would usually be hungry again two hours later. I couldn't understand it as my portion size was quite generous. After trying this hack and predominately going for savory options in the morning (my go-to is a side of veggies accompanied by two eggs on toast), I find that not only do I feel better, but I do not constantly feel the hunger nagging me as I go about my day.

Give it a try and see for yourself!

Hack 3: Save Up Your Sweets for Dessert

We've all been there. It's 2 p.m., and you feel a gurgle in your stomach after not eating for a couple of hours. You want a little nibble between meals, not something big, but something small and tasty. (That gurgle is a sign that your empty digestive tract is cleaning its walls.)

So, you go and reach for a little chocolate bite (or maybe a few). This is where this next hack comes into play. Instead of having that chocolate right then and there, take it and eat it after your next meal, and perhaps pick a savory snack. You might be wondering, *Ok, Morgana, but what difference does that make if I eat the chocolate after a meal versus as a small snack?* Let me explain.

When we are done eating, our organs keep working for about four hours. We are in what we call the *postprandial state*[12]. In this state, digestion takes place, and molecules are sorted and stored from food. Blood rushes to the digestive system, hormones rise, and some systems (like your immune system) are even put on hold!

Some systems become activated, however, like your fat storage. This is the largest hormonal and inflammatory state, and with our three meals per day and two snacks, we spend 20-24 hours of our day in this state. It's important to note that when we are not in our postprandial state, our insulin comes down, and we can go back to burning fat. (And we want that.)

In prehistoric times, people didn't have the luxury of being able to eat all day—quite the opposite. That means they had to possess something called metabolic flexibility[13]. This means that they could switch between burning glucose for fuel and fat for fuel quite quickly, depending on the availability of food. And it is a way to improve your metabolic health now by eating bigger meals and lessening your snacks.

Intermittent fasting is even proven to aid metabolic flexibility and train the body to switch between fat and glucose burning (but please consult

---

[12] Postprandial state: after food is ingested, this state occupies the digestion process and absorption of nutrients.
[13] Metabolic flexibility: ability to adapt in changing circumstances in metabolic demand.

with a nutritionally-informed doctor or dietitian before attempting intermittent fasting to see if it is right for you).

Now, if you add that chocolate to your dessert after your meal, you won't cause a midday glucose spike, and you will give your system a little break to properly digest your meal and burn fat. If you are hungry, opt for a fiber-rich snack!

Hack 4: Add Vinegar Before Meals

Vinegar is fermented alcohol. When taken before meals, it has been shown to enhance weight loss and reduce visceral fat, as well as slow the arrival of glucose into the bloodstream.

Acetic acid (acid coming from citrus fruits) is also beneficial as it gets into the bloodstream, penetrates the muscles, and speeds up the production of glycogen, which is a more efficient uptake of glucose.

A classic vinegar that I drink diluted in a large cup of water every morning before breakfast is apple cider vinegar. Another trick you can use is to add balsamic vinegar to a salad before you eat your main meal. This ultimately flattens glucose curves and curbs the amount of insulin produced by the meal that you are about to eat.

Even if you want to have oatmeal for breakfast or a simple pasta for lunch, try this hack and have some type of vinegar source before digging into those bare carbs.

I have a friend who was recently diagnosed with type 2 diabetes. His name is Aiden, and he was shocked to find out about all the dietary changes he would have to make (he was a huge lover of pasta, pizza, and sweets and not a huge fan of big protein portions or vegetables in general).

His doctor advised that every now and again, should he desire some carbohydrates to also drink some apple cider vinegar beforehand so that his glucose levels don't get out of control (please consult a doctor for your specific case before trying this if you are diagnosed with diabetes).

This little hack has proven to be a lifesaver for myself, my clients, and friends, who are only human, and sometimes we just want a little bit of simple carbs in our lives.

Hack 5: After You Eat, MOVE

As we established at the beginning of this chapter, our bodies use a lot of glucose every second to power our actions and bodily processes. Two things can happen once glucose is in our system.

If we are sedentary, glucose will peak and overwhelm the mitochondria, leading to glucose spikes. Or, if we use our muscles, it moves glucose from the intestine to the bloodstream to be immediately used and burned. (The harder a muscle is told to contract, the more energy it needs from glucose to be expended.)

If exercise is performed within 70 minutes (the time of a peak glucose spike) after the time you've eaten, glucose levels will even out without increasing insulin levels. And, the longer you work out, the flatter the curve you will create.

When I first heard about this trick, I decided to try it out. I would usually save my cleaning and household chores for after breakfast (which included vacuuming, sweeping the floors, and cleaning the stairs).

Usually, after lunch, I go on a midday walk to get out of the house between coaching calls. Or I will head to my dance studio and teach for a couple of hours. After dinner, I will either take a walk or do a set of squats to get that booty growing and muscles using that glucose.

Within two months, I had lost three pounds by isolating and trying this one hack. When glucose doesn't sit around in your liver or in your fat storage as glycogen but is used right away, it can have wonderful effects.

Additional Small Hacks

Although the five listed above will do more for your blood sugar than you know, these extra tips are useful to keep in mind. First, when you wake up, try to drink 8 oz (1 cup) of water which will aid blood sugar management, as well as eating breakfast within 90 minutes of waking to avoid hypoglycemia, especially in the luteal phase of your menstruation cycle (days 13-28).

For slow burners, keeping carbs at 30g for breakfast is useful as well (roughly two slices of whole wheat bread). This gives your system an adequate amount of glucose to work with without overdoing it. Eating lunch within 3.5 hours of breakfast also avoids hypoglycemia and its effects.

Now, do fruits have fructose? Yes. But are they the enemy? No. Fruits are still a useful source of vitamins, minerals, and antioxidants. The best fruit options that keep glucose levels steadier than others are berries, citrus fruits, and small, tart apples.

Similarly, even though alcohol does raise glucose levels, there are some that are better at keeping glucose levels steady. There are all types of wine and spirits: gin, vodka, tequila, whiskey, and rum. It is usually the mixers to these alcohols that have high sugar contents, and mixing them instead with sparkling water, lime, or lemon juices will allow you to have a drink every now and again. It should be noted, however, that beer does cause large glucose spikes due to its high carbohydrate content.

When it comes to cravings, we all know they are a b*tch. We've all been in that scenario where your body is crying out for something specific, whether it be sweet or salty or sour or tangy or meaty or carby. Whatever it may be, here are some tips to help those pesky cravings.

First (and you might not like this one), you can try waiting 20 minutes for your liver to contribute glucose to your bloodstream and for the craving to subside. I know it's a bit dull, but it is an option. Or, you can also resort to several craving killers. These include drinking licorice root tea, adding coconut oil or collagen peptides to coffee, drinking peppermint tea, chewing gum, or taking a walk.

Lastly, when finally eating something, or even walking in the grocery store and purchasing your food items, if sugar is listed on the top five ingredients on a nutrition label, it will indeed cause a glucose spike. Use the hacks listed in this section to avoid those spikes and eat what you love in peace.

Glucose Themes

You have successfully completed the first section of getting to know your body better. Congrats! (You have just gained a lot of knowledge, so I mean it when I say congrats).

We have learned about the four different types of sugar (starch, fructose, sucrose, and fiber), and their effects on the body. We have also learned in more detail about how they are metabolized and how they affect our glucose spikes.

Flattening these spikes will flatten insulin spikes and yield many positive benefits including decreasing cravings, entering "fat-burning" mode, lessening high and low dips of energy, and as we will later see, it will further help our other bodily processes.

To flatten these curves without taking away our beloved carbs, it was suggested that we eat in the correct order as a first step. You know how it goes: fiber, protein and fat, then our delicious carbs.

We also suggested to go savory for breakfast when possible, and to save those sweet bites you desire for snacks as dessert options once your body has adequate fiber levels. Adding vinegar before meals is another great tool, especially if you want to jump in straight with a heavy carb-centered meal (apple cider vinegar diluted in a glass of water is my usual go-to).

Lastly, going for a walk or performing some exercises after meals are great ways to use up the glucose that was just ingested without it getting stored in the liver and potentially in fat stores.

Please remember, we are only human. You do not have to use each hack with every meal. Otherwise, you will drive yourself crazy. You have the knowledge and can apply it accordingly based on the current meal and scenario.

This is the first step toward better health without restricting any foods! (Hello, fad diets, look-y here.) Your blood sugar is involved in many other bodily processes, and, as you see, it will also impact your hormones. You will begin to see the patterns and ripple effects throughout the interconnectedness of your body as we move through this book.

Let's explore it.

CHAPTER 3

HACKING YOUR HORMONES BACK INTO BALANCE

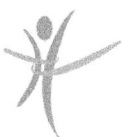

*"Balance is the perfect state of still water.
Let that be our model. It remains quiet within
and is not disturbed on the surface."*

—Confucius

Hey, hormones ... I've got a lot of questions for you. I mean, what's with the random crying, energy dips, emotional outbursts, and occasional fatigue? WTF. And you've got some explaining to do regarding why I get that huge pimple on the day of a really important meeting and why my internal thermostat is switching from being constantly cold to feeling like a boiling radiator some days of the month!

In this next chapter, we will discuss those handy **hormones** and delve deeper into the **endocrine system.** The endocrine system is made up of various glands that secrete a type of hormone that regulates a particular function in your body. It is these hormones that are in control of all of these problems mentioned above—from your energy levels, physical and mental activity, to your mood, to setting your body temperature, to metabolizing your food and determining your fertility.

It is such a large topic it honestly deserves its own book. But we will try to tackle the main ideas here so you can get a sense of the role your hormones play in relation to your other bodily systems.

For the purposes of simplicity and gaining a general understanding of your endocrine system, we won't discuss menstrual cycles. Our main focus will be understanding your hormones and their interactions with your organs and blood sugar.

First, complete the checklist below to see if you might have a hormonal imbalance and should check with your healthcare professional.

Hormone Symptom Checklist

Please tick the box that correlates with your symptom. If you have more than three of these symptoms, you should pay attention to several of the tips at the end of this chapter.

- Acne ☐
- Constipation ☐
- Mood swings ☐
- Bloating ☐
- Fatigue ☐
- Irregular/heavy periods ☐
- Stubborn weight ☐
- Subcutaneous fat ☐
- Low libido ☐

The Endocrine System

The simplest way to think of a hormone is that it is a little messenger molecule that travels around your body (via your bloodstream), telling your organs what to do. They work like supervisors in a company, giving directions and receiving information about how things are running.

Your hypothalamus[14] is the start of your endocrine control center. Your estrogen[15] and progesterone[16] receptors (two important hormones in women) are also found in the hypothalamus, as well as in the cardiovascular system and the kidneys.

This control center receives information from the bloodstream about concentrations of various hormones, and it will either send a releasing or inhibiting hormone to the pituitary gland[17] to send out or stop the flow of hormones. This gland lines up with your nose at the base of your brain and can be thought of as the CEO of the company, as it tells all of your other glands what to do.

Once hormone concentrations are received as signals in the brain, they communicate with other glands such as the thyroid[18], parathyroid[19], pancreas,[20] adrenals[21], and ovary glands,[22] with a different hormone for each.

---

[14] Hypothalamus: the area of the brain that controls hormones to give information related to body temperature, heart rate, hunger, and mood.
[15] Estrogen: a hormone that plays a role in the sexual and reproductive development in women.
[16] Progesterone: a steroid and sex hormone that plays a role in the menstrual cycle of women, as well as pregnancy.
[17] Pituitary gland: the controlling gland of the body.
[18] Thyroid: butterfly-shaped gland located at the front of the neck that secretes hormones.
[19] Parathyroid: this gland lies behind the thyroid and produces the parathyroid hormone which regulates calcium and phosphorus levels.
[20] Pancreas: an endocrine gland that regulates blood sugar and secretes insulin.
[21] Adrenal gland: located on top of both kidneys that help to regulate your metabolism, immune system, blood pressure and response to stress.
[22] Ovaries: small oval-shaped gland located on either side of the uterus. They produce and store eggs and make hormones responsible for reproductive health.

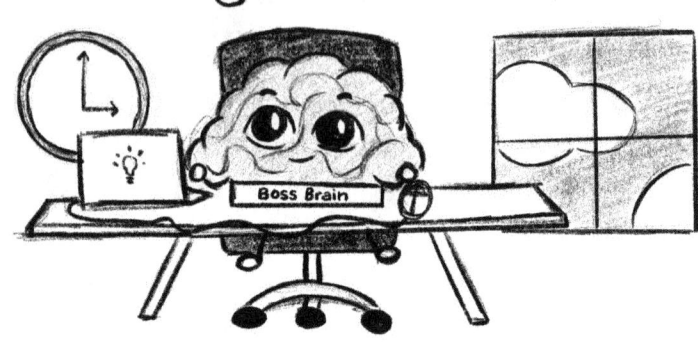
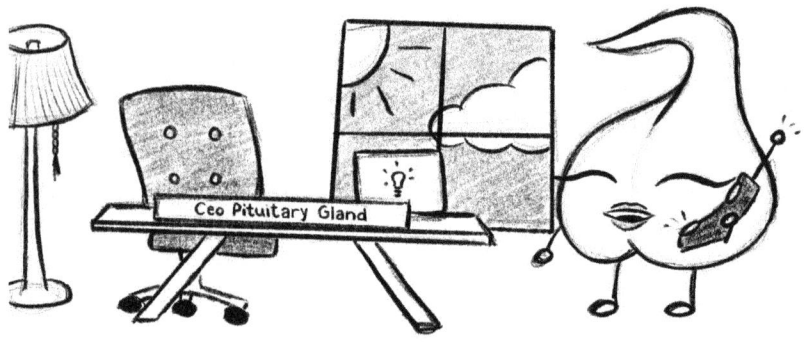
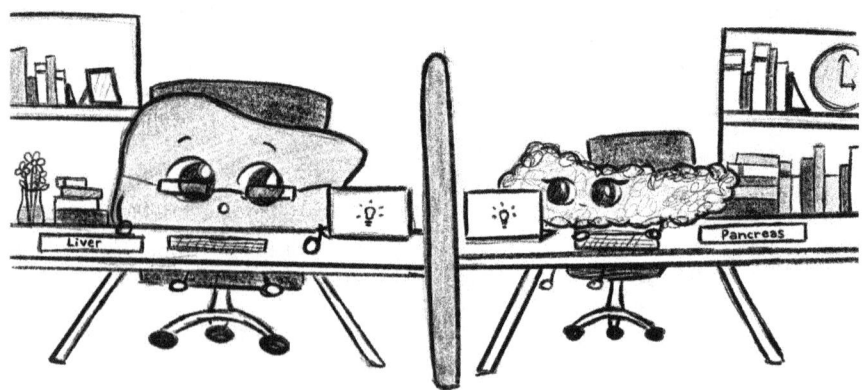

As hormones try to get the body back in balance, they can overcompensate and create other imbalances. It is amazing that they can self-regulate; however, our dietary and lifestyle choices play a huge role in their well-being.

As your hormones perform and aid in many roles, the easiest way to think about them is to break them down into subgroups for different functions. Alisa Vitti's book, *WomanCode*, labels these five groups as:

1. The blood sugar group
2. The stress group
3. The metabolic group
4. The elimination group
5. The reproductive group

The **blood sugar group** will sound vaguely familiar from the previous chapter, and now we will add hormones to the topic to connect the dots of our bodily processes. The pancreas handles this group.

As we know from above, when we ingest large amounts of glucose, our pancreas releases insulin. Our liver, however, is also involved in another process. The liver is responsible for breaking down estrogen that has been used and helping it leave the body.

If the liver is constantly trying to convert glycogen back to glucose because of low blood sugar (due to any of the difficult diets mentioned above), it is going to have less energy to eliminate excess estrogen.

This lingering estrogen leads to hormonal problems such as adenomyosis[23], endometriosis[24], and more. It is then advised to use food to stabilize blood sugar levels and not rely on our liver to do the job so that it can focus on its predominant role of getting rid of excess estrogen (see the next tips section in this chapter).

---
[23] Adenomyosis: when the tissue of the uterus begins to grow into the surrounding muscle wall.
[24] Endometriosis: disease where the lining of the uterus grows outside of it.

Ahhh, the **stress group**. The one we probably each put a little too much strain on. In ancient times, the fight-or-flight stress response was good because it helped keep us alert and ready for danger and was used occasionally.

Nowadays, we live in states of chronic stress due to the fast-paced nature of our lives. This puts a heavy strain on our bodies and leads to heart disease, stroke, insomnia, weight gain, fatigue, challenged fertility, and a decreased sex drive.

When stressed, the adrenal glands (which sit on top of each kidney) will release cortisol.[25] Cortisol serves several functions. It can help reduce inflammation, increase the body's metabolism of glucose, control blood pressure, and of course help in response to danger. This is regulated by the pituitary gland (the main supervisor of all the glands).

Now, as you are reading this, I want you to take note of your body. Unfurrow your eyebrows, unclench your jaw, let your tongue release from the top of your mouth, release any tension you are holding in your legs, and take a deep breath in. Notice how much tension we unconsciously carry? Destressing methods are vital for adrenal health, and these will be detailed in the tips section of this chapter.

Next, we come to the **metabolic group**. This group is regulated by the thyroid and parathyroid glands located at the base of the neck. This group is so sensitive that nearly one out of two women suffer thyroid issues at least once in their lifetime. Stress, smoking, fasting, alcohol, and certain medications can all affect thyroid levels, hence why it is so sensitive.

The thyroid gland will secrete the thyroid hormone, which is known for determining your BMR.[26] It sets your heart rate and regulates blood pressure, breathing rate, body temperature, and the rate at which your cells

---

[25] Cortisol: the "stress" hormone released from adrenal glands to initiate bodily processes to combat stress.
[26] BMR (basal metabolic rate): the number of calories your body burns at rest.

consume oxygen. In our early years, the thyroid also aids the development of bone growth and the development of the brain and nervous system.

The parathyroid group secretes the parathyroid hormone, which regulates calcium and phosphorus levels in the body. Your bone and tooth development are dependent on this gland. The hormone calcitonin[27] signals the parathyroid to redistribute some of the calcium to avoid low calcium levels, which can lead to dangerous conditions like osteoporosis.

Fourth, we have the **elimination group**, the body's natural detox-er. Fun fact, when you go to poo, your hormones are also present in that stool sample (a lovely image I just created, isn't it)?

We don't only excrete hormones via our stool; our skin (the largest organ in our bodies) also secretes excess hormones when we sweat.

Let's back up a second and get a detailed look at this system. This elimination group is aided by the liver, large intestine, lymphatic system[28], and skin. This group does not secrete hormones, but as the name suggests, it eliminates them.

This is vital to our health as a buildup of hormones in our bodies becomes toxic to our health (for example, a build-up of estrogen can lead to aiding tumor growth).

The liver breaks down hormones into tiny molecules to be excreted by the colon. Our bodies have a functioning automatic system that far surpasses any technology out there! However, when our systems get out of balance, the system can no longer work efficiently (imagine if a tire on your car deflated. Technically, you can still drive, but you won't get very far)!

Issues like chronic constipation and GI disorders like IBS can lead to a build-up of hormones in the body without a way to get rid of them unless

---

[27] Calcitonin: hormone the thyroid gland makes to regulate calcium levels in the body.
[28] Lymphatic system: group of organs and tissues that fight against infection and keep a healthy fluid balance throughout the body.

they are addressed. As mentioned, skin sweat removes these toxins as well. When your stool exit is compromised, it will affect your other system of elimination.

The lymphatic system is comprised of tissues and fluids that ward against infection and maintain fluid balance in the system. When there is a hormone overload situation in your body, you will notice your sweat will smell different (and not a good different). We will tackle tips on how to best serve this system to avoid hormone toxicity, and not just by adding some more deodorant.

Lastly, we come to the **reproductive group**. This group involves a conversation between the pituitary gland, the ovaries, and the hypothalamus. Based on the levels of estrogen and progesterone hormones that the ovaries secrete, the hypothalamus will tell the pituitary gland to send either the follicle-stimulating hormone or luteinizing hormone, coinciding with the follicular or luteal phases of your menstrual cycle.

This affects fertility, mood, water retention, energy, and sex drive. Based on what week of the month it is, your body, as the beautiful and complicated creature it is, has different hormonal concentrations. Hence, the conversation back to the brain is so important!

This reproductive group is complex and deserves its own book (maybe an idea for the future). However, we will keep the topic simple and focus on strategies to serve the five groups best. But first, we need to understand what can lead to blockages in our system.

Endocrine Disruptors

Endocrine disruptors are chemicals that aggravate the production, release, transport, metabolism, or elimination of the body's natural hormones. This can occur through the air we breathe, our water intake, soil quality, food, and consumer products. They can mimic the natural hormones our bodies make, causing an overproduction or underproduction of the naturally occurring ones.

These chemical compounds with their science-y doodad names like xenoestrogens[29], BPA[30], and phthalates[31] are becoming increasingly seen in the food items we buy (mostly in the processed food items, but they have also infiltrated our whole foods system as well). The three compounds listed above have estrogen-like qualities and effects, which can lead to reproductive issues.

An article titled "Sex Hormones in Meat and Dairy Products" mentions six hormones approved by the FDA for use in food products. They include three naturally occurring hormones: estradiol[32], progesterone, and testosterone[33], and three man-made ones: zeranol[34], trenbolone acetate[35], and melengesterol acetate[36]. These hormones are mainly added to the dairy and meat sector.

Manipulating growth hormones can lead to an increase in the production of other hormones in our body, like insulin, and we have just spent all that time learning about how to flatten our insulin curves. Damnit.

The article also details that pregnant cows whose milk is ingested have higher levels of estrogen and therefore can cause an overabundance in our systems. It is great that there are many milk and dairy alternatives available today, as they can help us steer clear of these hormonal issues.

However, coming to the meat sector, many hormones are pumped into animal bodies to make them larger and more attractive to the consumer eye when purchasing.

Their feed is also changed, usually to GMO corn, which can alter their chemical compositions further and add further toxicity to our diets. An

---

[29] Xenoestrogen: a chemical mix that resembles estrogen very closely that it is able to bind to estrogen receptor sites, with an increased chance of complications.
[30] BPA (bisphenol A): chemical substance used to replicate plastics and resins.
[31] Phthalate: a group of chemicals used to make plastics more durable.
[32] Estradiol: hormone made in the body by the ovaries.
[33] Testosterone: primarily male sex hormone.
[34] Zeranol: used to destress cattle with estrogen-like effects (growth-stimulant).
[35] Trenbolone acetate: used in livestock to increase appetite and growth.
[36] Melengesterol acetate: suppresses menstruation in livestock for food and breeding purposes.

example of this is that a chicken's diet does not usually consist of corn; however, if you went to a chicken farm nowadays, I bet you would see some corn feed being munched down on.

This is a huge reason I went plant-based. Once I was diagnosed with adenomyosis, it all made much more sense that I had an overabundance of estrogen in my system. Although the doctor merely prescribed me birth control pills, he did mention that I should look into diet alternatives.

So, I took matters into my own hands and did the research. Once I found that dairy and meat had so many additional hormones, it greatly influenced my decision to go plant-based and use predominantly dairy alternatives (I still eat cheese, though; I'm only human).

I became my own experiment after I had read up on plant-based diets, and after one month without meat and dairy, my face became so much clearer. I was amazed I could walk outside without makeup for the first time since my teen years, and my confidence skyrocketed.

My client Esther was a die-hard meat eater. She, too, was diagnosed with adenomyosis and struggled with acne and uncontrollable weight gain. She had hoped to have children in the future and worried about her condition.

When we started to work together, I suggested she cut down on the meat to a level that we agreed felt comfortable to her. When she limited eating meat to twice a week for dinner, her acne began to clear. She also experienced some weight loss.

According to her, "I have never been more surprised at how quickly I could lose weight and clear my face. Once I understood my problem properly and the tools to combat it, it made so much sense, and I was so relieved!"

Here's why: estrogen promotes fat storage. When estrogen levels are balanced, a healthy fat level can also be achieved. Once Esther began to see the results, she became completely plant-based and even took it a step further to become vegan. She no longer craved meat and loved how she looked and felt.

Stress is another endocrine disruptor. Anxiety affects our body's signals. Feedback from the hypothalamus to the pituitary and adrenal glands is lessened, which changes digestion, moods, libido, and energy levels.

Further, when we are stressed, we are activating our sympathetic nervous system. In this system, glucose is used for energy, and the body will hold onto its reserves as a safety mechanism. It's kinda like the movie *Inside Out* (if you haven't watched it, you are missing out). The movie is based on emotions living as characters inside a young child's brain, driving their behavior. Now imagine if stress was at the control panel—all the time. The control panel would constantly be on red alert, and all systems would be shut down.

We ideally want to be predominantly living within our parasympathetic nervous system, or as it's also called, the "rest and digest" system. (This is when calmness takes over the control board, the red alert is switched off, and systems go green). You can switch this by destressing and slowing your heart rate down.

Another little fun fact about our friend Mr. Stress is that he also causes inflammation in the body, which throws off your hormones. Fad diets tend to have this effect, as there is usually too much sugar, fewer nutrients, and increased codependency on alcohol and caffeine.

When I first learned about these disruptors, it made sense logically. Then, I began to listen to my body more and more. I can now tell when my system is dealing with excess hormones, and I know how to deal with it. I have, as we call it, become "in tune with my body." And I aspire for you to have this as well.

Your body is a wise vessel, and it knows what it needs. You just need to be clever enough to listen. This is why I firmly believe that learning about our systems is the first step. The second step is to get useful tips to help in areas you might need.

Endocrine Tips

Stabilize Your Blood Sugar

Sounds familiar, eh? (Sorry for my Canadian-ness.) Well, it is, in fact, the first tip on how to better balance your hormones. Your body perceives mismanaged blood sugar as a stressor, which tells the adrenal glands to send out cortisol and adrenaline[37]. This is proof that all the various bodily systems are intertwined and how when one is off kilter, it affects all the other processes.

Low blood sugar states cause the body to seek out large amounts of food, as it is in "starvation mode." Vitti quoted several studies that found that when blood sugar levels were normalized, activity in the prefrontal cortex kicked in, and the desire for junk food decreased.

The five tools listed in the glucose section of the book will help get blood sugar levels back on track. Additional tools include the use of cinnamon and/or drinking peppermint or rooibos tea.

*Chill the F*ck Out*

Dude, why so stressed? (This is coming from the most tightly wound person ever, believe me.) But seriously, it is so important to take care of your adrenals. Adrenal fatigue is the result of built-up stress. The symptoms include tiredness, acne, weight gain, insomnia, depression, increased susceptibility to colds and infections, and high sugar cravings.

The first indicator of adrenal fatigue is the infamous "night owl syndrome." Those people who call themselves night owls typically can't fall asleep until very late in the night and have trouble waking up.

---

[37] Adrenaline: natural hormone released in response to stress.

This is a result of adrenal surges: a redirection of blood to muscles to increase energy, being pushed later into the night when they typically should be between 8 a.m. and 8 p.m.

To get back on track, it is important to know what sets off adrenals. They include low blood sugar, irregular sleeping patterns, a lack of regular orgasms (as funny as it may seem, they are a huge stress reliever), financial troubles, and long commutes.

The best de-stressors include:

- Yoga
- Meditation
- Breathing exercises
- Getting in charge of your schedule
- Journaling
- Cleaning up your home space
- Eating more whole foods and less junk food
- Simply slowing down

Yoga (I recommend hot yoga) is an amazing, uplifting practice that focuses the mind during the class and clears chakras[38] (energy centers). Meditation is another practice that is amazing at shifting energy and focusing the mind.

Breathing exercises are a powerful practice to add to your morning routine. They allow you to focus and be present in that moment so you can continue your day in a calm state (allowing Ms. Calm to take over the control panel).

---

[38] Chakra: energy centers in the body, usually in large nerve bundles and are found around major organs.

Organizing your schedule also has powerful effects on your mindset once you can feel good knowing that everything is booked and written down in a calendar. Journaling your thoughts when you are stressed allows for the release of that negative energy onto the piece of paper. This transference of energy will leave you feeling lighter and more at peace.

Cleaning up your home space is one of my personal favorites. Perhaps it is just me, but if my home is disorganized and messy, I feel my thoughts get messy (a bit weird, I know). This creates stress for me, and when I reorganize and put everything in its place, I feel as though I have done an internal sweep of my brain.

We will get to the energetics portion of this book, but eating more whole foods will give you more energy than junk food, and it won't stress your system out with metabolizing the extra sugar and salt.

Lastly, simply slowing down has got to be the most obvious but perhaps the most difficult. You don't need to do everything right now, sister. I've been there, and I've done that.

There will forever be one million things on your to-do list, and it will get done in due time. Take care to pace yourself and set boundaries over your schedule. (As an added tip, adding holy basil to your tea will help mitigate stress.)

One of my friends, Jessica, is a maximalist like me (probably why we get along so well). She is ambitious and an overachiever, and there is nothing wrong with that.

However, when we saw each other, her comments were laced with remarks about fatigue and low energy, sentences accompanied by complaints about small amounts of weight gain and not being able to fall asleep due to her overactive mind.

The first tip I suggested to her was to meditate at the start of her day. She now wakes up and sets a meditation podcast for 10 minutes and is able to start her day off with a clearer mindset.

She then took control of her schedule, prioritizing certain tasks and not getting bothered or stressed if others didn't get done that day. Lastly, she switched her habit of turning to chocolate whenever she was feeling overstressed and instead found comfort in eating sliced mango (which, when eaten, calms neuroreceptors in the brain).

All of a sudden, Jessica had heaps more energy, and her mindset was calmer, which allowed her to overcome her adrenal fatigue.

Support Your Organs of Elimination

No, they don't need a shoulder to lean on. That's not what I meant by support. What they need are certain key nutrients so they can clear out hormones from your system to prevent overload.

Let's start bottom-up. Healthy bowel movements are medium brown, curved, and smooth. It is important to inspect them from time to time as they are indicators of what is going on inside of you. Fiber, B vitamins, and artichoke leaves offer great nutrients for supporting bowel movements.

Constipation can be solved by increasing your water intake, eating more of certain fruits like prunes and apples, eating sweet potatoes, and decreasing processed foods. To avoid future complications, try to steer clear of laxatives. They can create dependency on them to have any sort of bowel movement at all, which is not a sign of a healthy working digestive system.

Your skin sweat is another organ of elimination that expels toxins. Your skin is the last place a hormonal issue will occur. If acne or bad-smelling sweat starts to occur, it is an indicator that a hormonal problem has been brewing for a while (I wish someone had told me that sooner).

To ensure skin toxins are expelled, try exfoliating a few times per week. Frequenting saunas two times a week is another way to get your sweat on and a deep clean of this important organ. Another great way to flush toxins from the skin is to change the shower temperature from hot to cold a few times, as it causes your cells to contract and expand, pushing out any stubborn toxins.

The lymphatic system is designed to sweep up metabolic waste, including dead cells and excess fluid from organs, and put them into the bloodstream. It also allows for the free flow of progesterone, which is designed to balance estrogen levels. (As we know now, unbalanced estrogen can lead to many hormonal issues and cause serious symptoms.)

When working efficiently, it directs white blood cells to invaders to fight viruses. When it is compromised, the white blood cell fluid will attract more viruses and bacteria, leading to increased rate of infections.

To keep the lymphatic system healthy, fill your diet with hearty vegetables such as cabbage, cauliflower, broccoli, Brussels sprouts, and kale. Adding lemons to water is another added nutrient support, as well as eating dill and caraway seeds.

The lymphatic system relies on the movement of the body to circulate its fluid since it has no pump of its own. That's why it's vital to get daily exercise, stretch regularly, and practice deep breathing.

You could even spoil yourself with the occasional massage. In this way, you're still moving toxins out, but you're getting to relax at the same time! Just be sure to drink plenty of water afterward to help flush those toxins out of your system.

Summary Chart:

Bowel Movement Aids	Skin Elimination Aids	Lymphatic System Aids
Consuming fiber	Exfoliate	Eat more hearty vegetables
Adding B vitamins, sweet potato, prunes, apples, and artichoke leaves to diet	Go to sauna or steam rooms 1-2 times per week	Increase water intake and add lemons to water
Drinking more water	Shower with changing temperatures	Try adding dill and caraway seeds to diet
Avoiding processed foods		Daily exercise and stretches
		Massages
		Deep breathing

Try Dairy and Gluten Alternatives

As discussed in the previous section, dairy is loaded with estrogen. Vitti, in her book *WomanCode*, states that it accounts for roughly 60-80% of the estrogen consumed within the American diet (p. 196). **Gluten,** on the other hand, can cause inflammation of the small intestine.

However, as you are reading, it's important to remember that everyone is different. I am dairy-free, but I am not gluten-free or gluten-sensitive. I have experimented with going gluten-free; however, I feel no difference in my body on this diet change.

Sometimes, I will swap for a gluten-free alternative in a restaurant if what I'm ordering contains a lot of carbs (and could potentially overload my system), but for me, it is not an issue.

Many of my clients and people I know do have sensitivities to gluten and feel immensely better gluten-free. Celiac disease has become increasingly common; about 1% of people worldwide have this disease.

Restaurants and chains are becoming more aware of the conscious consumer and have many alternatives available on the menu. The same goes for grocery shopping, but it is important to test and experiment with what works well for you and what doesn't.

What to Do When Your Human Urges Arise

It's 9 p.m., and you order a pizza. You dig in. You take in all of that carby goodness and relish every moment. By 10:30, you are preparing to go to bed as you have an early working day tomorrow, but you feel full and uncomfortable. Try to drink 16 oz of water, take a probiotic, or go for a walk to help your stomach compensate for that drastic blood sugar increase (which will push your adrenal surge later, making it difficult to fall asleep).

You're getting ready for a party. Down goes one cocktail, then another. And then your BFF suggests you do shots before you leave. You feel the burning sensation down your throat and know that you will feel that bad boy tomorrow.

Alcohol can impair the functions of the glands we discussed that release hormones. About blood sugar, it also stops glucose production while alcohol is being metabolized. Beyond that, it raises the body's cortisol levels during and after consumption. So, what to do?

It's important to rehydrate to flush your system. Try taking one glass of water for every drink of alcohol as a rule of thumb. Taking a B-vitamin supplement will also help replenish lost nutrients, as will drinking something with electrolytes to properly rehydrate. Doing hot yoga is another great way to allow for the alcohol toxins to be excreted through the skin and to destress.

Normal Problems, Normal Solutions

If you struggle with either (or a combination of) acne, fatigue, bloating, mood swings, and sugar lows, try these tricks to combat them and get your hormones back on track:

Acne

- Drink more water
- Eat more leafy greens
- Reduce dairy intake
- Reduce sugar intake
- Reduce animal protein

Fatigue

- Drink more water
- Decrease sugar and caffeine (the opposite of what you'd think)
- Determine what is stressing you out and use coping strategies outlined in the "Chill the F*ck Out" tip section.

Bloating

- Drink more water
- Eat more fennel
- Reduce salt
- Reduce processed foods

Mood Swings and Sugar Lows

- Increase consumption of sweet vegetables like beets and sweet potatoes
- Eat more whole grains
- Drink more water
- Increase healthy protein
- Reduce sugar and caffeine

So, did we notice any recurring themes? Coming in first place is "Drink more water"! Hydration is key to restoring hormonal imbalances. Another important note is to reduce processed foods, which will automatically lower sugar and salt intake and decrease these hormonal issues that I know plague many women from time to time.

Hormonal Themes

As we wrap up this important bodily process, I ask you to think back on what you learned. First, we learned that hormones are secreted by various glands in our bodies, and they are our body's messengers. They communicate with the hypothalamus to guide and dictate the release or inhibiting action of the glands.

We also saw just how big a role our hormones play. The five groups mentioned (blood sugar group, stress group, metabolic group, elimination group, and reproductive group) all work to manage bodily functions.

These can be disrupted by environmental circumstances such as bad air, water and soil quality, and the addition of synthetic and naturally occurring hormones to the food industry. This can overload the hormonal system and cause imbalances.

Stress is another disruptor that can upset the flow of hormones, as well as those "fantastic" fad diets we have been talking so much about. To combat these disruptors, we discussed how to manage blood sugar levels as a first step.

To take it a step further, de-stressing methods were outlined, followed by tips on how to better our systems of elimination. Assessing how the body copes with dairy and gluten are other great tools to try and, if needed, steer clear of.

Now that we have a deeper understanding of our hormones and blood sugar levels, shall we step into the world of the gut-mind connection?

Yes, we shall.

CHAPTER 4

TRUST YOUR GUT

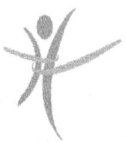

"Intuition is the essence of being a woman."

—Anais Nin

Not too long ago, my friend Jenny went through a really bad breakup. It was a long relationship that ended dramatically. After the breakup, she was consumed with memories, stress, and grief. She would cry whenever she was at home (and sometimes at work, much to her coworkers' dismay).

She knew she should be eating, but she didn't feel hungry. She would attempt breakfast sometimes but could barely eat anything. This went on for a week and a half until her emotions began to clarify, and her stress began to fade. Almost magically, as she started to feel better, her hunger began to return.

Stress is truly a powerful indicator in our body and is an example of how our emotions can halt normal, automatic processes that can disrupt our appetite, digestion, and cravings.

Have you ever wondered why you suddenly get the shits when you're just minutes away from presenting a project to your boss? Or why do you get constipated when you're bombarded with loads of work?

Your body can't tell the difference between the stress of actual danger and the stress of having too much to do in too little time. In the case of constipation, it's saying, "Let me just hold off on digesting this breakfast, and let's divert our energy to deal with the impending danger." Even if the perceived "danger" is too many emails at once, your body's response is to redirect that energy.

This is exactly how your emotions can activate or deactivate your digestive system. That's the gut-brain connection, baby!

Gut-Brain Connection Symptom Checklist

Before we learn more about this topic, take a second and check the boxes of the symptoms that apply to you. If you experience three or more of these symptoms, you should prioritize your gut health and use several of the tips toward the end of this chapter.

- GI issues ☐
- Mood swings ☐
- Depression ☐
- Anxiety ☐
- Panic attacks ☐
- Constipation ☐
- Diarrhea ☐
- Cravings ☐
- Emotional eating habits ☐

Gut-Brain Connection Explained

I know what you're thinking ... how in the hell are my gut and brain so linked that everyone keeps talking about their connection (but not really explaining it)? Well, you would be surprised by how many similarities your gut and brain possess.

First, your gut is studded with endocrine cells containing up to 20 different types of hormones (hello, hormones ... connecting those bodily processes), which can be released into the bloodstream.

To illustrate the gut-brain connection, we're gonna use an example from your childhood. Stay with me here. Did you ever find a pole or pool floaty or random object that should not be anywhere near a child's mouth (yet you put it there) and tried to communicate with your friend through it? Well, I did. Maybe I had an interesting childhood. Who knows?

In this example, the gut is on one side, and your brain is on the other. The pole or floaty or object represents the nerve cables that run between our brains and guts.

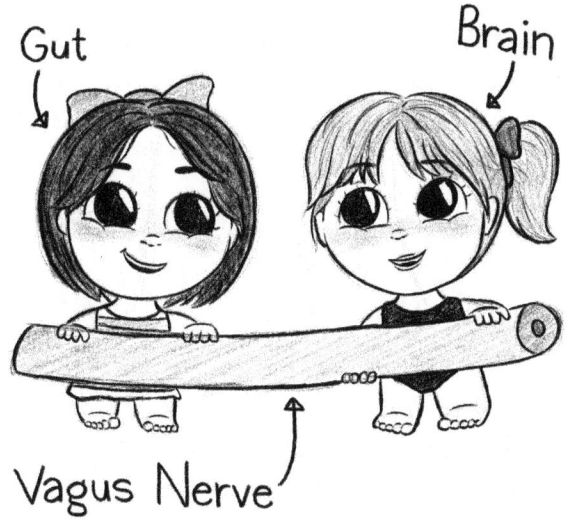

There is one nerve cable in particular that you might have heard of: the **vagus nerve**. This nerve runs from the brainstem to the abdomen, connecting the gut and brain. It aids in digestion signaling and forms what scientists call the **gut-brain axis**.

Those hormones we just discussed, as well as inflammatory signaling molecules, transfer information about the gut's well-being to the brain through this nerve cable. So basically if your gut is being loved on and is doing well, the gut will whisper "all is good," into the pipe and it will make it to the other side where the brain is listening with the message intact.

If there is something wrong, perhaps some form of food intolerance, lack of pre and probiotics, sunlight, whole foods, etc., that message will get broken by the time it reaches the brain.

Imagine if a pesky younger sibling of yours jumped into the pool and yanked the tube out of your hands mid-message. (I'd be pretty upset, I don't know about you.) That is often what happens with our body when our gut health is out of alignment.

Emeran Mayer, gastroenterologist, neuroscientist, and author of *The Mind-Gut Connection: How the Hidden Conversation Within Our Bodies Impacts Our Mood, Our Choices, and Our Overall Health*, explains that neurons sit inside the gut lining outside of direct contact with the gut.

With the help of the cells that line the gut, a scan of the gut microbiome can be done and communicated with those neurons to then give a complete breakdown to the brain (like you have to do when you give your boss your weekly reports).

There is also another linkage between the two. Inflammatory molecules that immune cells (living inside of our gut) produce are called cytokines[39]. Ok, I know it's a complex word that's a bit confusing. Don't

---

[39] Cytokines: small proteins crucial for the growth and activity of immune and blood cells.

panic. All you need to know is that these cytokine molecules can cross the gut lining, enter blood circulation, and reach the brain. It's a way our gut signals inflammation to the brain.

Although essential, it's not exactly desirable to have communication channels regarding inflammation. It's almost as if rude intruders interrupted mid-game and wanted to take part in sending the message.

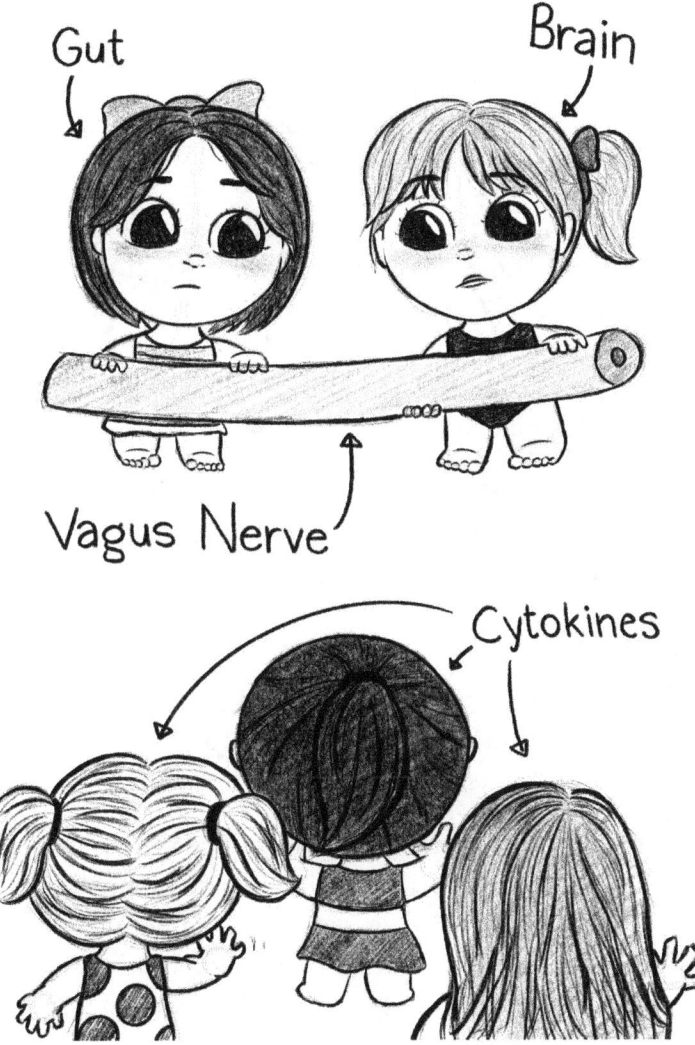

As we can see, there are multiple pathways through which information is communicated from the gut to the brain. The two work cohesively to send messages and responses to one another.

Another important key factor in this topic is serotonin (which is super important for your happiness)! Serotonin involves the chemical messages between the nerve cells in the brain and other parts of the body and is important for regulating mood, sleep, appetite, and normal intestinal functions.

The gut is the largest **serotonin** storage organ in the body, with 95% of its total residing there (talk about a sensory organ). Thus, the gut and brain communicate similarly and share many of the same molecules.

I hope to show you that the two are more alike than we give them credit for, and perhaps emotions do play a role in what and when we eat. We will begin to discuss this by showing how gut feelings are created when we feel a certain way, whether it be stressed, anxious, happy, depressed, etc., and how they are then stored in the brain and affect our decisions related to appetite and cravings.

First, we need to understand more about our **gut microbes** to gain deeper insight into this organ before we can even think about discussing our ever-so-complicated emotions.

Gut Microbes

Gut microbes, or our microbiota, refer to the bacteria, fungi, and viruses as a collective that reside in the gut. I know it's a bit gross to think about, but we need all these microorganisms to be healthy!

They function through obtaining nutrients from their hosts (us), and in exchange, they help keep the gut in balance by providing us with essential vitamins, metabolizing digestive compounds such as bile acids produced in the liver, metabolism, and immune system regulation, and detoxifying foreign chemicals that our bodies haven't encountered before. It's a give-and-take relationship, you could say. They are also responsible for digesting dietary fiber and complex sugar molecules that our digestive system can't break down or absorb on its own.

They are so vital to the gut that you might also be surprised that our microbiota gathers information about our food and environment every millisecond! Isn't it insane how much our bodies look out for us?! This information is then fed back to the brain to make calculated decisions and automate bodily processes.

Here's where it gets interesting. Mayer wrote that the location and closeness of our microbes let them listen to brain signals that detail how stressed we are and our happiness, anxiety, and anger levels.

Ok, back up. *How in the hell?* I wish I could tell you I'm joking, but I swear I'm not. The two organs are sooooo connected, it's unbelievable.

Ever remember feeling stressed about a big presentation and feeling butterflies in your stomach? Yep. Gut-brain connection.

Or, if you've ever gone through a terrible breakup, do you remember not being hungry for a week or two? (Been there, done that … it's what we call the post-breakup body.)

That is all related to how closely linked our brain and gut are and how deeply our emotions play a role in what we choose to eat, when we eat, and how often we eat.

Diet, lifestyle, and antibiotics affect the connection sensitivity between the gut and the brain, and to better this connection, I will go over some tips toward the end of this chapter. (You want to be sure in your friendly childhood game in the pool that the right message will reach the end of the tube!)

However, the well-being of our gut microbes depends on the foods we eat and have been programmed to prefer during the first few years of life (more on this in the "Starting in the Womb" section). It is very difficult to increase microbial diversity, even through the aid of probiotics, kimchi, and sauerkraut superfoods you may have heard about.

Their diversity stays relatively stable, and how we build them up in the early years plays a big role in our long-term health. So, mamas, pay attention to the coming sections not just for your health but also for your child's future and well-being.

High-animal fat diets have been shown to increase the negative bacteria found in the gut, and diets low in plant-based fiber result in our gut microbes beginning to feed on their own mucus lining—the one that separates the gut from the immune system and keeps bacteria out of other tissues. Yikes.

If the lining is being eaten away, it can become dangerous and lead to severe symptoms such as inflammation and infection. The lining even has defense mechanisms comparable to an electric fence in the event of opportunistic bacteria.

All in all, I think you can see why when your mom told you to eat your veggies as a kid, she had your best interest at heart. This shows how important diet is to maintain one's health and to keep bodily processes running properly.

Digestive Forces

I felt it inappropriate to speak so much about the gut and not talk in detail about the digestive process that occurs in our bodies, especially since our goal at the end of this book is for you to have a general, deeper understanding of all of the bodily processes that go on.

As a heads-up, you might feel like dozing off in this small section as it can get slightly technical, but I will do my best to liven it up for you.

So, as you may already know, when you eat, your teeth grind food into smaller molecules, and nutrients are beginning to be absorbed in the mouth. These smaller molecules travel down the esophagus, where it makes its first pit stop in the stomach. Your stomach is filled with hydrochloric acid[40], and grinding forces help further break food up into even smaller particles. Oddly enough, writing this makes me hungry.

The gallbladder and pancreas then prepare the small intestine by injecting bile to digest the fat from the food, as well as a variety of digestive enzymes. They are then broken down into nutrients that the gut can absorb and transfer to the rest of the body.

The muscles surrounding the intestines then perform muscular contractions called peristalsis[41]. This moves the food to the small intestine, where nutrients are absorbed. Further contractions move the food to the rectum. Stool is then excreted as the digestive process takes its final bow. Cue the curtain. And it takes its final exit.

However, for its encore, between meals, we have something called a migrating motor complex. This essentially sweeps everything not dissolved from the digestion process to the colon every 90 minutes. This is why intermittent fasting is beneficial for some (again, experiment and see if it works for you), as it gives the organs involved in digestion a break for several hours, and the cleanup crew can do a couple of sweeps to make sure they got all of the mess (they can't do their job if more food is incoming).

Whew. You made it through your eighth grade science class recap. My apologies for those technicalities, but I hope you can visualize the route your food takes in your body. Now, let's connect those dots to the topic at hand—gut-brain connection.

---

[40] Hydrochloric acid: the acid that breaks down food in the stomach and enzymes that split up proteins.
[41] Peristalsis: involuntary contractions of muscles throughout the digestive tract.

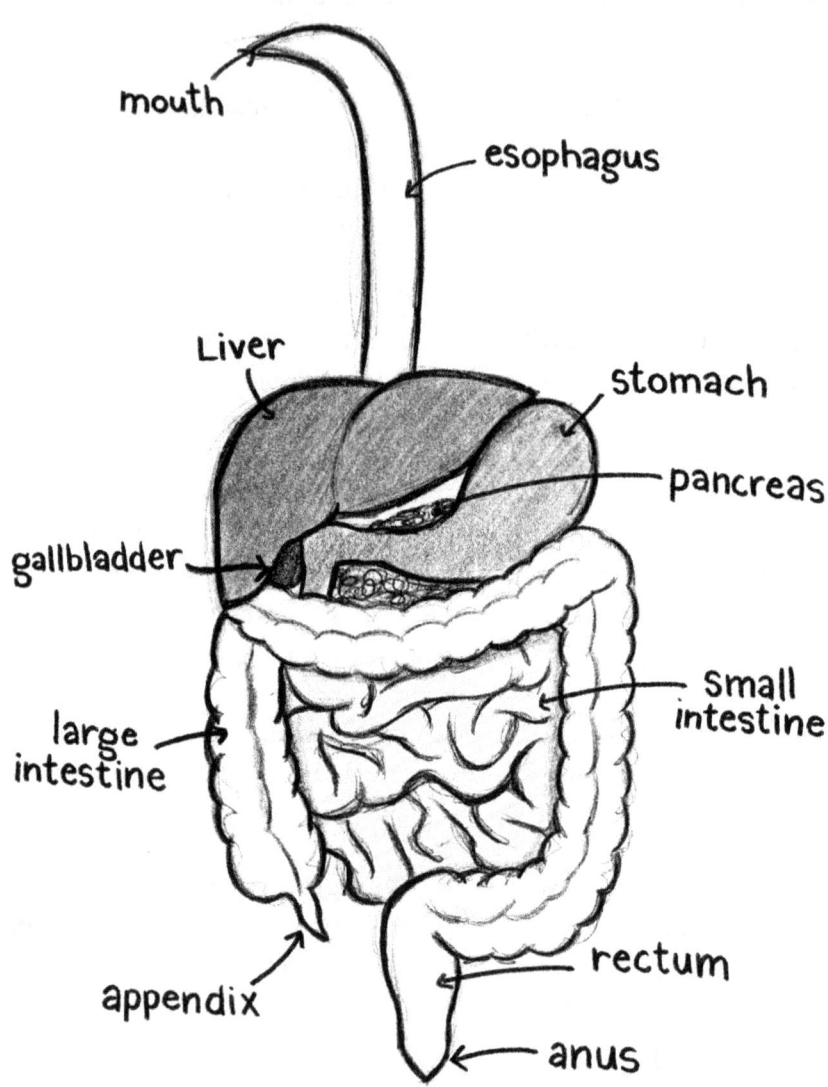

Image of the organs involved in the digestive process.

Managing your digestion is the work of your enteric nervous system. This involves 50 million nerve cells that are wrapped around the intestine, spanning from the esophagus to the rectum. It operates independently from the brain; however, the emotional component of our brains can automatically halt and interfere with these automatic processes, thickening the plot of our gut-brain connection.

To better understand this connection, I think it's time we talked about the OG—the big bad boss—the one, the only … the brain.

The Brain

This is a biggie. I'm not going to lie. I am a bit overwhelmed as I write this, as I am no neuroscientist. So, I humbly state that the points I will illustrate do not paint a large enough picture of the **brain**. They will merely try to show the emotional contexts of our development in relation to the gut; however, there are many other neurological processes that take place that would best be portrayed by someone who has extensively studied the brain for years. Nevertheless, I'll take a swing at it.

First, the brain has two sides: the left side and the right side. The left side is responsible for language and logic, whereas the right side deals with creativity and intuition.

However, the brain's primary job is to process information and regulate the body. This works in tune with the gut as gut messages have been detailed in the section above, and now we will discuss a bit further in how the brain regulates those messages.

Your brain is constantly being fed information from all the systems we listed, not only your gut. It is also keeping up with your hormone levels, glucose spikes, how your organs are doing, impending danger, what outfit you should wear to that festival you've been looking forward to, and the exact curve of the smile of your crush. It's a 24/7 job being you.

Once it is fed information about your gut, it will send hungry or full hormones out to signal whether it needs some food or not (however, the processed food industry can trick this basic process). It will also influence which cravings and nutrients your body needs and wants.

As we have seen, all of our systems are interconnected. So, let's say your blood sugar is spiking constantly; more hungry hormones will be sent out via the brain.

Or, perhaps you have too many toxins in your body, and your brain has to tell your liver to chill with the hormone processing and instead focus on transforming those toxins into less harmful substances.

Or, maybe you have candida growth in your gut, which is signaling to your brain to seek out other forms of starch and sugar. It's in constant two-way communication. I hope your "body talk" is made clear because now we are going to add emotions to this fun mix and show their impact on your bodily processes (and yes, they do indeed impede on your bodily functions; they are not only in your head)!

Emotions play an enormous impact on how our body functions. In relation to this, I feel it important to mention that in the brain, there exist neurons called von Economo neurons[42].

These are large, highly connected neurons that help us make intuitive decisions. We usually say, "Listen to your gut" or "Trust your intuition." Well, you're not far off. It's crazy that when we say this, we are really referring to our gut-brain axis, as gut messages are communicated to the brain and play a role in these intuitive decisions. These neurons lie on the right side of the brain, as well as receptors for social bonds.

---

[42] Von Economo neurons: neurons located in the right brain that are linked to aiding in intuitive decision-making.

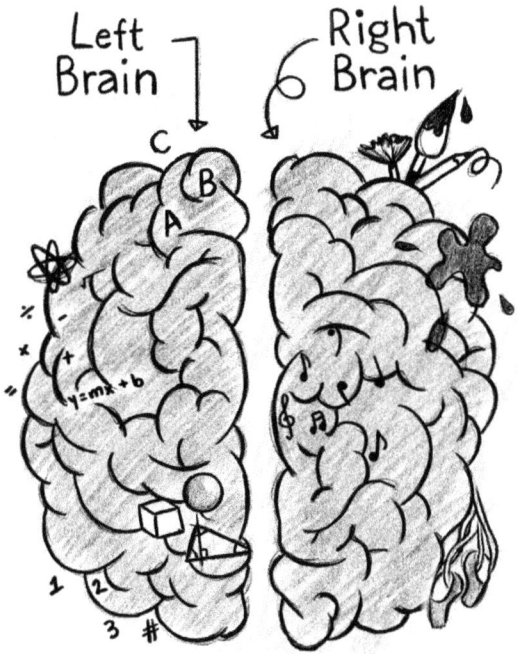

Depiction of the right versus left side of the brain and what each is responsible for.

The enteric nervous system alters the gut environment and manages digestion by contracting acidity, fluidity, secretions of digestive fluids, and mechanical contractions of the GI tract.

Our emotional reactions also create and inhibit these responses. Stress and anxiety have huge physical ramifications. They can alter gut contractions and the rate at which your digestion occurs. It even affects how your blood flows through your body!

For example, stress can cause constipation as the cardiovascular system reroutes oxygen-rich blood from the gut to the muscles to prepare to fight or flee, which is an inhibiting example.

On the flip side, emotion-related brain circuits will send signals to the stomach and intestine to empty to get energy that might be needed for action. We definitely don't want constipation or diarrhea to be a regular occurrence!

Those with IBS or functional bowel issues like constipation and diarrhea will feel these emotional effects take on physical inabilities and problems. It is said to go as far as IBS being treated through antidepressant drugs (there are much better lifestyle tools to manage depression and stress than medication, just saying)!

Even simply working on bettering your gut health (which we're coming to soon, I promise) will help with your feelings of depression and anxiety (if you experience them, of course).

This topic will be further detailed in the next section to point out the scientific impact our emotions have on our gut and digestion.

How Are Your Emotions Involved?

As we now know, there is such a thing as the gut-brain axis, and the two organs are connected in various ways. We also know that somehow emotions play a key role in the signaling that goes back and forth.

Let's take a closer look at this theme to really see and understand the central role emotions have in the gut-brain connection.

When a big emotion is experienced, the brain releases stress hormones such as cortisol and adrenaline, and nerve signals are dispatched. There are then two different reactions that can take place. Either they will stimulate gut functions or they will inhibit them. After the emotion has passed, the digestive system will switch back to normal.

Although we have covered this in our discussion, I felt it important to show you what role your brain has in this process (if you are as analytical as me). This explains so much about emotional eating, or the lack of it, and how large of a role our emotions play in our food choices from a scientific perspective.

Your gut helps determine the intensity, duration, and uniqueness of your emotional feelings through the gut microbiota (you really are what you eat). Anything that modifies or disrupts the microbiota (such as stress, diet, antibiotics, and probiotics) can affect how responsive it is to these emotions.

Let's say you have just failed a course, and perhaps you have been eating that crappy university diet for way too long, filled with sugar, caffeine, alcohol, and processed foods. Your reaction to this news and the emotional intensity of what you feel will be worsened because of the bad nutrition choices you made. You can achieve clarity and calmness through a balanced diet of whole foods. If you want to feel better, you need to treat yourself better.

If you are a PMS girlie, you'll need to give yourself extra attention. The week leading up to your period, when you get those sugary carb cravings, take good care of yourself. Indulging in those cravings will actually make your symptoms so much worse! It is much better to swap out other types of whole-food carbs to curb those cravings. Sweet potatoes are an excellent example, and the beta-carotene found in them will also help support your reproductive hormones. Win-win!

Coming back to our emotions and our understanding of their role in our body, on an average day, cortisol can help maintain proper fat, protein, and carbohydrate metabolism, as well as keep the immune system in check.

Stressful situations cause a dramatic increase in the corticotropin-releasing factor [43] (CRF). CRF regulates the amount of cortisol produced by the adrenal glands.

It is interesting that environmental stimuli can affect this stress and set off this reaction, even with negative memories felt in certain locations or attached to certain foods.

---

[43] CRF: initiates a response in the brain that releases cortisol.

Let's take the classic example of eating a tub of ice cream after a breakup. Stress and anxiety levels are high at this time, and eating that tub of ice cream has now created an emotional memory toward this food. You might begin to associate this food choice whenever you experience any kind of stress in the future as a coping mechanism.

The same goes for locations. If you are out to dinner with your spouse and you get into an argument, there could be a negative memory and stressful feeling associated with that location, which sets off a chain of stress reactions in the body when revisiting it. (Make sure you don't fight at your favorite restaurant.)

Our emotional operating systems allow us to respond instantly, and these programs have been shown to be genetic. Emotional core memories and how they influence the gut are inherited and influenced by events we experience early in life (but also don't blame your parents; they were doing their best).

If you experienced trauma as a child, you may experience exaggerated gut symptoms as an adult (learn more about this in the next section). This linkage between emotions and the gut goes as far as the documentation and studies performed by Mayer that illustrate how people with autism, depression, and GI disorders have very different gut microbiomes than that of the average person.

Science has actually come super far to now have learned that fecal transplants (super gross to even think about, I know) from a healthy person into someone with a GI disorder or someone who has autism drastically help their condition! And don't worry, this isn't one of the tips coming up. There are definitely less invasive and gross ways we can help the gut heal.

These points provide scientific explanations for what you might have experienced or felt regarding emotional eating or not being hungry in cases of extreme stress, as well as the digestive consequences.

In illustrating this connection and process, you can begin healing your emotional connection with food and gain a better understanding of it. Now that you know your emotional brain influences your appetite, sensitivity, and mood, you can perhaps go on to heal your emotional side and your emotional state when eating to maintain or build a healthier relationship with food, rather than again unknowingly trying a fad diet to get better eating habits.

As we have discussed, it doesn't work in the long run. Your newfound understanding can open many avenues to healing that perhaps you hadn't thought of before.

Starting in the Womb

I'm sure you are well aware of how important the shaping of a child is in their early years, but maybe you have only thought about it from a behavioral perspective.

What if I told you that the first 2.5 to 3 years shape a baby's gut microbiome for a lifetime? That is crazy, and it is so influential that I thought it important to include this section here so that you can help your future or perhaps current kids shape healthy gut microbiomes.

This is done through interactions with the world, including social influences, diet (breast milk quality), and the chemicals found in the food they are consuming. They can impact their immune cells, hormones, and nerve endings.

Breast milk bacteria are influenced by the food the mother consumes, which is then transferred to the child. (Apparently, my mom really craved donuts when she was pregnant with me, and here I am, 25 years later, with a sweet tooth—thanks, Mom.) Studies have also shown that the longer an infant is breastfed, the larger its brain and, therefore, the more cognitive development it will have.

Mothers, keep pumping! In comes the next generation of super babies! No, but all jokes aside, this is an important connection for families to know so they can make the best choices for their children.

There is also a connection between breastfeeding and influencing a baby's emotional and social development due to the hormone release of oxytocin experienced by both the mother and child while nursing. In other words, this will deepen your relationship with your child and also make you both that much happier.

However, if you have chosen to go another way, I want you to know, Mama, that your choice is valid. Don't feel guilty over doing what you feel and know in your core is best for you and your child. So if breastfeeding is not in your repertoire, to hell with it!

Another important connection is that during birth, the mother's vaginal microbes are the first seed for the baby's gut microbiota. Children born via C-section are shown to be missing important flora in their digestive systems later in adult life and may suffer from GI issues. One of my friends was born through a C-section (the mother didn't have a choice), and now, later in life, she has colitis. Is this completely random? I think not, especially since she grew up around whole foods and home cooking!

Mayer reported several studies on monkeys that depicted maternal stress in the womb and how it altered a baby's gut microbiota, and the same held true for human babies. Researchers studied monkeys in Thailand from gestation to the first two years of their offspring's lives and found that mothers who were stressed due to food shortages showed the effects in their offspring. They had a weakened immune system and a slower learning time for their motor abilities.

It is also shown that stress changes a human mother's vaginal bacteria, which is then passed on to her children during birth. Hopefully, the illustration between the birthing, breastfeeding, and first years of the child's development of their gut microbiomes are made clear and vitally important to be looked after to set them up for healthy futures and to promote you to make the best choices for your family.

So what can you do? Obviously, you can't be completely stress-free for nine months of your pregnancy. It is very difficult on a woman's body. On the other hand, working with a professional health coach (like me!) or finding out the best self-care and stress-relieving practices for you are so important for you and your baby's well-being.

You may have also heard of a little something called a woman's intuition. Well, it is scientifically a real thing. Women have been shown to have greater sensitivity to the brain's salience and emotional arousal systems connected with their physical feelings. This is because women store their memories of physiologically painful and uncomfortable states from situations such as menstruation, pregnancy, and childbirth. Why we do that, I'll never know.

This makes us more sensitive than men in this department. I mean, we knew that already, didn't we? So, it all stems from the mother and her well-being to obtain optimal vaginal bacteria and breast milk quality, as well as her intuition stored from her gut experiences. Now, ladies, we won't be perfect. You can't provide the best environment for your child 24/7, and that's good. Sometimes, kids need to be exposed to bacteria to build their immunity and learn how to find their own stress-coping practices. Just do your best, so you feel good and nourished, and your baby will be A-Ok.

As we move on from this section, take this knowledge with you and use it to influence your family in a positive way, and we will commence the discussion of food addiction and further our topic of diets.

Food Addiction and Diets

What if I told you dieting wasn't about "self-control"? What if it had nothing to do with how much willpower you have or your discipline level? Sure, I mean, there is a place for that. But, many times, diets not being followed have nothing to do with one's discipline level and everything to do with regular bodily processes dictating appetite and satiety.

We are often made to feel guilty or out of control by those who oversee our diets, or it is rather self-inflicted, or both. Whichever it is, I just want you to know that there is only so much one person can do when succumbing to intelligent marketing campaigns and food restriction.

We will learn about how our appetite is dictated so you can better understand this process and make better choices. I remember many a time when I was restricting calories and trying not to eat for the majority of the day, and then feeling so guilty when I would come home and eat everything in sight—including a tub of sugar-laden vegan ice cream (as I had associated this food with my saddened state and it became the norm for me in my fad dieting phase). It doesn't have to be this way! There is a way toward a healthy appetite and falling out of food addiction.

How much food you eat is controlled by three related systems in the brain. First, your appetite is controlled by the hypothalamus. The second system involved is your dopamine[44] reward system, designed to give you pleasure and satisfaction. This also motivates you to "hunt" and obtain your food, so take your spear and head to the grocery store. Lastly, there is an executive control system in your prefrontal cortex which can override the other two control systems. This can occur from food memories (like remembering that beautiful tiramisu cake you ate in Italy, which causes you to taste-test every tiramisu that crosses your path so you can try to relive the same experience). This is very dangerous nowadays, as food is very, very palatable.

All that added sugar, salt, and fat is designed to target your brain's reward system and make you desire it. This can allow the executive control system to take over, regardless of whether you are full, and make you eat the food being advertised or marketed.

---

[44] Dopamine: molecule that acts in the brain to provide satisfaction, pleasure, and motivation.

Hitting this point further home, high-fat diets can numb the satiety response (your feeling of being full) at the gut and brain levels. Many processed foods create this level of food addiction and make you unable to stop eating until it is done.

Imagine stopping at half the can of Pringles. You can't, huh? I know I used to not be able to. I had to finish Every. Last. One. This is a sign of food addiction, the uncontrollable urge to eat palatable foods, even when you're not hungry. This can also consume your thoughts and further spark your addiction.

A client of mine, Amanda, suffered from food addiction. She did everything right. She exercised daily and ate three healthy meals a day. During those meals, she could stop when she was full.

However, she had stubborn fat around her waist, and she wanted to get rid of her uncontrollable snacking habit. She was a lover of chips and soda (I mean, aren't we all), but she used to tell me, "Morgana, I can't stop until every chip is finished and the soda bottle is empty."

This was not a once-in-a-while occurrence. It was every day. Sometimes multiple times a day! We worked from an emotional perspective to identify her food and emotional connections, and I suggested healthier snack options that wouldn't upset her control system and get it out of whack.

She found satisfaction in snacks like homemade granola, baked potato wedges, and veggies with hummus, and by fueling her body with water instead of sugary drinks, she lost her belly fat within one month.

She also loved preparing the snacks herself, as she could use her creativity, get away from processed and artificial ingredients, and de-stress in the process. Once you learn the triggers, it becomes much easier to make better choices for yourself.

It's important to note where the calories are coming from that lead to food addiction. Many books and documentaries I have used in my research have all touched on the Standard American Diet, or S.A.D., as it clearly is. More than 35% of the American diet calories come from animal fat sources, which contributes largely to the problem of overconsumption.

When conventional animal products are consumed, an immediate inflammation response occurs in our bodies. This starts in the gut and can spread throughout the body toward the brain, including to those regions that control our appetite.

This constant low-grade inflammation has contributed to the start of many diseases. As we have learned together, there are many pathways through which the gut and brain communicate. Once there is inflammation, hormones travel through the blood and communicate with the gut and brain.

The information that is allowed through depends on the thickness and integrity of the gut mucus layer lining and its permeability. It's kind of like breaking the chocolate barrier in a Magnum ice cream container (can you tell I used to eat a lot of ice cream)?

Stress, inflammation, a high-fat diet, and certain food additives can make the barriers leakier, leading to a loss of communication toward satiety and appetite.

Imagine if you bought a tub of that beautiful ice cream, cracked open the jar and found that the chocolate was barely there and broken into already? I imagine you'd be pretty upset and might even ask for a refund. After all, that crunch and those chocolate bits are kinda the whole point. *Anyways, Morgana, refocus. Quit the ice cream talk.*

Food emulsifiers[45] have a similar effect on the gut. These detergent-like molecules found in many processed foods help mix two things together that normally don't mix, like oil and water, for example. These are found in many sauces, candies, and bakery products.

---

[45] Food emulsifiers: food additive that helps mix two substances.

Food emulsifiers can disrupt the mucus layer in the gut, giving gut microbes easier access to the gut lining, which can lead to many infections and low-grade inflammation. Artificial sweeteners are another common additive in the processed food industry, and they have the same effect as a high-fat diet, causing inflammation and decreased communication between the gut and brain.

If you have ever felt or are currently feeling that you can't control your eating patterns or that you dream or fantasize about certain foods, that is not normal eating behavior. You don't need to feel guilty, restricted, or out of control.

There are tools to get you back on track, and now you have a further understanding of how your appetite is regulated, so you can look at that can of Pringles square in the face and tell it to f*ck off.

Tips for a Happier Gut

Add Fermented Foods to Your Diet

Fermented foods are an excellent diet addition. Foods such as pickles, sauerkraut, pickled onions, and kimchi introduce healthy bacteria to your gut. As well, they are great when eaten first in a meal as they act in the same acidic way as vinegar to balance glucose levels throughout your meal. You are, as they say, "killing two birds with one stone."

Decrease the Animal Products in Your Overall Diet

As we have covered, animal products are high in fat and can lead to overconsumption and food addiction, as well as chronic low-grade inflammation in the gut, disrupting communication with the brain.

Animal products don't refer to just the meat obtained but also by-products such as milk, dairy, and eggs that also contribute to inflammation. Eating more whole-food and plant-based foods in your diet will have a tremendous impact on decreasing inflammation in your gut, and you will experience less bloating and fatigue. You will also be able to become more in tune with your appetite and satiety.

Help Your Future and Current Children or Help a New Mother

Learning information on how to start a healthy gut microbiome for your children or for the child of a new mother you might know is priceless information! It is so vital to how they will digest food as adults and whether or not they will have gut issues in the future.

Ensure that mothers minimize stress when possible while pregnant and opt for vaginal birth methods rather than C-sections. Likewise, mothers might want to research vegan alternatives while pregnant to not pass any toxins found in meat and animal products onto their offspring (as mothers have the ability to rid their toxins ingested by passing them on to their children in the womb).

There are many amazing books and tools out there to help you on your vegan pregnancy journey if that is the route you want to take. Whichever direction you decide to take your pregnancy, do what you feel is best for you and your future child. You have a beautiful intuition; trust it.

Eat Happy

I know this sounds weird, but it is actually so important, and it is something we will touch on in the next chapter. Eating in a negative state throws your system out of balance by introducing stress hormones to the gut. This causes inflammation and makes it leakier.

This domino effect continues to your brain and, of course, the control processes there. Enjoying meals together in a happy social setting is something your gut microbes love! When you eat happier, your body responds in a similar way, and you can reap those benefits. Stay tuned for more on this.

Add More Color to Your Plate

Aim for two to three colors per plate. Every color is designed to give your body a different nutrient, and the more nutrient-dense your diet is, the happier your gut will be. Think reds, oranges, yellows, blues, purples, and, of course, greens.

Reds are amazing anti-inflammatories. Oranges give your body some beautiful beta-carotene to help your reproductive organs. Yellows are excellent pre and probiotics to boost your gut health. Greens give your body an abundance of different minerals that are targeted toward benefitting your heart health and circulation. Blues and purples are true brain food and can even help further your creativity.

Mother Nature gave us the medicine; we just need to be smart enough to take it.

Gut-Brain Themes

This section might have been a surprise for you. Maybe all of this time you have been picturing some imaginary gut-brain connection and have been surprised to find out that there actually are things connecting them including the vagus nerve, as well as the communication between the gut microbes and the brain.

The enteric nervous system also plays a key role. We have also discussed how your emotions have physical impacts on your digestion, either inhibiting or causing contractions in relation to stress or other deep-seated emotions. So perhaps next time, before you give that talk or presentation, you will opt for some de-stressing methods rather than rushing to the toilet directly afterward.

Inflammation is an important marker of stress and gut flare-ups. These signals are sent to the brain, and the result? GI disorders.

Additionally, starting in the womb was a key part of this chapter, as well as highlighting preventative routes that mothers can take for their children and for the betterment of their health during their pregnancy.

Appetite and its brain origins are another topic that was dissected to show the idea that willpower is sometimes not enough of a defense against the ploys of the processed food industry.

Again, these are good reminders of several of the beginning ideas we spoke about regarding processed foods and difficult diets. I hope that you try the tips outlined and document whether you see a difference in your bowel movements, brain clarity, emotions, and energy. Keep what serves you and forget what doesn't!

We will wrap all of these ideas up in a nice little bow soon enough to tie in these main themes and what actions you can take to better your bodily processes all at once.

CHAPTER 5

EATING FOR ENERGY

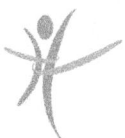

"True health infuses positive energy in the mind, body and spirit."

—Maximillian Degenerez

If you've made it this far, I want you to know that I appreciate you! There is a lot of technical jargon that I have tried to put into its simplest form, so you have a clearer understanding of our bodily processes.

Now, the next subject is energetics, and it is one that I hold near and dear to my heart, but I realize I might lose some readers at this point. Before we begin, I want to ask that you keep an open mind and think of food as a transference of energy to us (which it is).

The way I came to study this topic became instinctive. I always questioned why whenever I would eat certain processed foods like chips or chocolate bars, I would feel like crap afterward, although I liked the taste, and my dopamine receptors certainly enjoyed them as well. I would feel slow and sluggish not just for the rest of the day but for two or three days after that. I constantly thought about this conundrum.

When I began eating certain types of whole foods, I realized I had heaps of energy. I could go to dance training all day, come home and study nutrition-related subjects, and proceed to write this book. It was a complete mystery for me.

First, I rationalized that it had something to do with my horoscope or just that I had more sleep that day. Then, I got back in touch with what I was eating, and it all made sense. And I will make it make sense now for you too. Before then, let's do our usual chapter checklist to see if some of your symptoms align with low energetics.

Low Energetics Symptoms Checklist

Please tick the box that corresponds with your symptom. If you have ticked more than three, consider taking a closer look at some of the foods you are eating.

- Fatigue ☐
- Habitual eating ☐
- Constant need for caffeine ☐
- Low drive and purpose ☐
- Large dependence on processed foods ☐
- High levels of stress and anxiety ☐
- Depression ☐
- Stubborn weight ☐

All About Energetics

Our bodies are mostly made of energy. Even as you sit and read this book, your body is producing 100 watts of energy. Water has also been tested and proven to omit a *vibrational frequency*[46]. We are made of mostly

---

[46] Vibrational frequency: the number of vibration cycles one object completes in one second.

water and hold this vibrational frequency. The foods we eat, therefore, hold a certain amount of energy.

In physics, a vibration is defined as a periodic back-and-forth motion of particles as they move away from their equilibrium. Ew, I know, I have taken you back to your high school days of sitting in a physics class. I was not the brightest in physics (just ask my dad), but some things stuck, and some things I have to include (#sorrynotsorry).

Coming back to my mind-boggling question of why certain foods made me feel energized and why others left me feeling either the same or slower and sluggish is because of the level of vibration they omit. Processed foods are low in vibration and do not provide the body with adequate energy levels to perform at an optimal level.

It is proven that your body can heal and repair itself when the vibration is at a certain rate and frequency. But how do we get it there?

Note how I said that our *body* can heal and repair itself. If we give it the right tools and nutrients, it can heal a broken bone, repair a cut, clear your skin, resolve GI disorders, reverse growths, and do just about anything. So, the next time you are dealing with a symptom, don't head straight for that Advil. Try raising your vibration instead.

First, the easiest way is to prepare food with love and in a positive, energetic space. As sappy and corny as it sounds, it's true. Whole, living foods can alter and change their genetic structures to grow nutrients your body needs; however, they need the right positive environment to do so.

This is why it is great if you grow your own fruits and vegetables, as they provide tailor-made medicine for you, your spirit, and your body.

Foods that are high in vibration also exist. Those include:

- Organic fresh fruits and vegetables
- Herbal teas
- Herbs and spices

- Healthy oils like olive oil, avocado oil, and coconut oils. (Tip: using coconut oil when cooking enhances the nutrients of a food.)
- Nuts and seeds
- Fermented foods
- Raw chocolate
- Raw honey and raw maple syrup (the Canadian in me loves this)
- Legumes
- Whole grains like rice, quinoa, and buckwheat

Examples of low-vibrational foods include:

- GMO foods that have been chemically interfered with
- Artificial sugars and sweeteners
- Soda and high-sugar fruit juices
- Alcohol
- Processed foods
- Unhealthy seed oils like canola oil and rapeseed oil
- Foods that have been prepared via microwave or that have been deep-fried

Still don't believe me? Dr. Valerie Hunt released a YouTube video that details energy field images. She began by showing a dog and the energy that was omitted when it was reunited with its owner to give an example of what positive electromagnetic energies[47] to look for (still waiting for my boyfriend to gift me my own bundle of joy, Sigh).

Next, she showed a man eating a fast-food burger. He omitted no electromagnetic energy, perhaps because it wasn't a happy meal. Okay, I'm not a comic, so I'll stay in my lane. The next clip showed the same man

---

[47] Electromagnetic energy: waves of energy that range from long to short gamma rays.

eating fruit, and he had three times the electromagnetic energy radiating from him.

She then went on to explain in her science-y terms how negatively charged ions replenish and vitalize our energy fields, which refers to the high-vibrational foods listed above (anything that is on a shelf or has been pasteurized is referred to as a "dead food," meaning it has no life force).

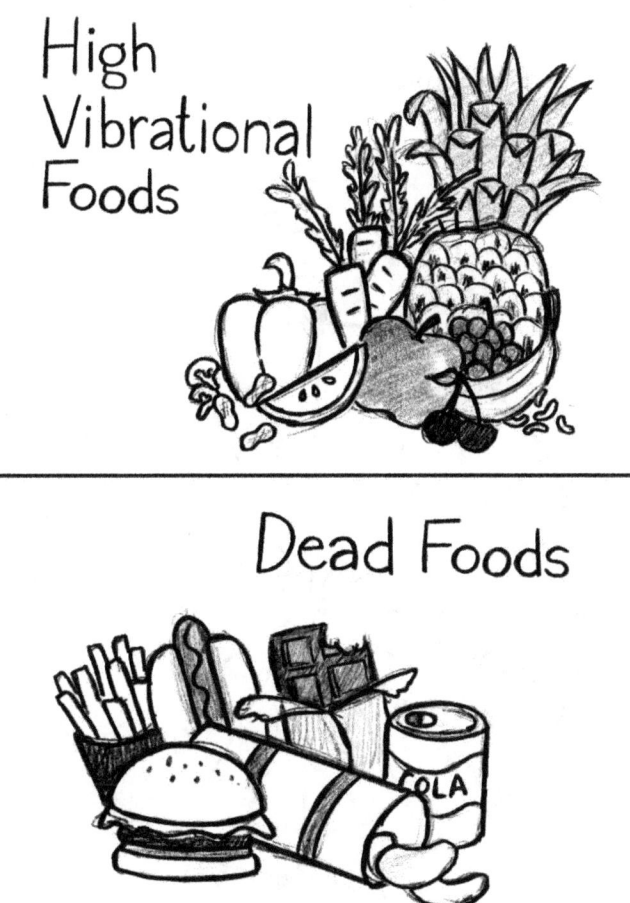

This even extends beyond food to our daily energies. Our process of living requires that we replenish our life force.

Nourishing Yourself Outside of Your Plate

Do you ever notice that you don't eat as much food when practicing yoga, watching a sunset, or even out in the fresh air for a portion of your day? This is because you are being filled with life force energy and do not require as much food to give you that energy transference.

The circle of life exercise, referring to primary foods (nourishment that comes from outside of your plate), is a fantastic tool I learned during my time at IIN. We will do it here together so you can see an area of your life you might want to devote extra attention to and be sure that you are not using food as a coping mechanism to fill the void in this area.

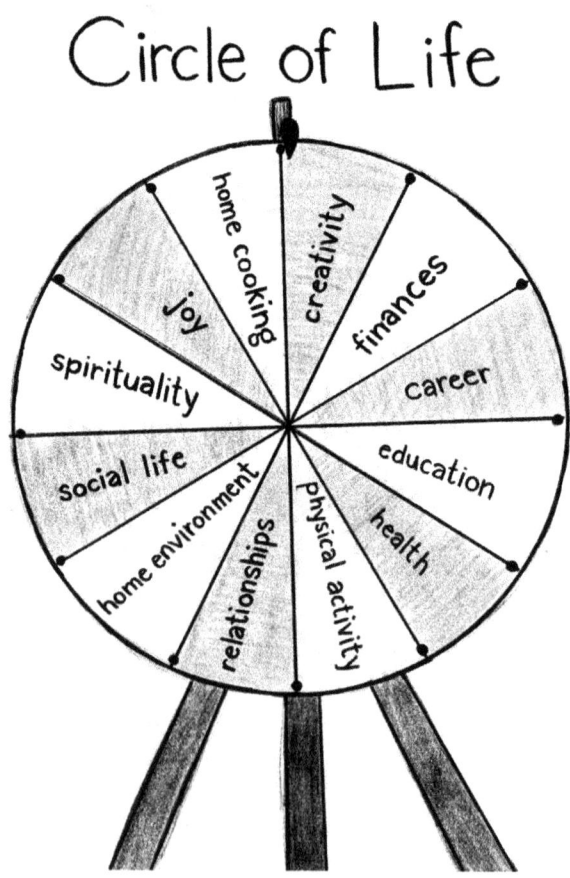

There are 12 categories in our general lifestyle. I will list them, and I want you to rank this category on a scale of 1-10 (1 being awful and 10 being amazing):

1. Creativity
   _____

2. Finances
   _____

3. Career
   _____

4. Education
   _____

5. Health
   _____

6. Physical Activity
   _____

7. Home Cooking
   _____

8. Home Environment
   _____

9. Relationships
   _____

10. Social Life
    _____

11. Joy
    _____

12. Spirituality
    _____

Take a second and see which category might need a little bit of extra loving. While this book won't go into a heavy primary food discussion, be sure to check out my next book to get answers in the area you are struggling with (currently in the works)!

Ask yourself what steps you can take to improve this area of your life and nourish yourself in areas other than your plate. (Use your inner baby Yoda!)

Returning to our vibration talk, even when you prepare and cook food yourself, you usually don't eat as much as you would in a restaurant because there, the food is less nutrient dense and doesn't hold the same vibration.

It's important to remember that good food helps you connect with who you are and allows you to tune into your inner guidance so you can manifest and think clearly.

The Power to Heal Naturally

Western medicine, all good intentions aside, is essentially a mushed-up chemical pile designed to treat symptoms. Notice my choice of wording there, "to treat *symptoms*," not the root cause.

Western medicine may hold the tools for the cure, but we will never know as, at the end of the day, the business goal is to have repeat purchases. What kind of profitable business would sell the cure knowing that there are other ways to ensure constant business?

Frank Lipman, a doctor turned holistic healer, cleverly put it as Western medicine playing whack-a-mole. A disease pops up, and they whack it with a drug, and then it pops up somewhere else. This repeats on and on until someone is taking so many different pills and suffering from their side effects.

I know I am bashing Western medicine. I don't mean to. It has helped many people worldwide, and many people involved in the health sector are well-intentioned in their purposes to help. However, Mother Nature has already provided us with natural cures.

In his book *Medical Medium: Life-Changing Foods*, Anthony William writes about how fruits, vegetables, and herbs have the healing powers to cure our ailments, with detailed descriptions for each food item. It is truly insightful.

He discusses the fact that plant foods contain two different types of water. The first, hydrobioactive water [48], replenishes the body, feeds the bloodstream, and keeps you going from an energy standpoint. Examples include coconut water or simply adding lemon slices to your water.

Let's do an experiment for a second. Pretend you are out on a hot day and absolutely parched. Now, imagine an ice-cold glass of (filtered) water. You also have a choice between the same water with lemon added this time. Which one are you reaching for? Biologically, our bodies know and crave the one that will bring us more hydration.

The second type of water is one that William discovered and has yet to be documented by scientists. It is called cofactor water[49]. It contains information to help restore your soul and spirit and support emotions. This cofactor water contains trace minerals, mineral salts, enzymes, and phytochemicals[50]. This is truly revolutionary, and it makes sense that illnesses would have cures readily available in nature.

This pertains to food **energetics** and how high-vibrational foods can indeed raise frequencies to combat illnesses. Let's take a look at an example of an apple.

---

[48] Hydrobioactive water: term suggested by Anthony Williams that suggests that this type of water hydrates the body more so than tap water.
[49] Cofactor water: the part of fruits and vegetables that holds spiritual information, according to Williams.
[50] Phytochemical: compound found in plants.

IBS is one of the most common gut issues nowadays. In walks the handy apple. Apples are naturally anti-inflammatory, increase digestive strength, and have weight loss properties. They are also the ultimate colon cleansers, picking up bad bacteria as they move their way down the colon.

Celery is another example of a powerful anti-inflammatory agent. It starves unproductive yeast, bacteria, mold, fungus, and viruses in the body and flushes these toxins out of the intestinal tract and liver. It also raises the hydrochloric acid in the stomach so that food digests with ease, along with restoring overworked adrenal glands.

Taking an example from the herb category comes the handy raspberry leaf. Let me tell you, ladies, this will become your new best friend. This herb balances a woman's reproductive organs and feeds the thyroid gland. It can go as far as preventing exhaustion after childbirth and can help protect against miscarriages. This herb is also powerful for men as it acts as a blood cleanser, detoxer, and hair grower.

This just goes to show that Mama Nature knows best. Next time you are thinking of taking a laxative, try an apple instead. Indigestion? Eat some celery. Cramps, ladies? Try raspberry leaf-infused tea.

Oriental Medicine Beliefs

The Chinese, specifically, follow ancient practices regarding food, energy, and healing. You may have heard of yin and yang (I'm sure you are picturing that white and black symbol in your head). Well, what if I told you that it also pertains to food and healing and that the Chinese eat to restore their **yin** and **yang**, as well as their **qi**, **blood**, and **essence**?

Yin is the water of the body, and when in harmony, it allows bodily processes to flow like a well-oiled machine. Yang is the opposite, naturally. It is the fire of the body, and all life processes require heat. If Yang is low, we cool down, and the metabolism slows.

Qi is referred to as the available energy of a person and food (hello food energetics). With the help of exercise, fresh air, acupuncture, and postural adjustments, can increase our Qi or energy availability.

Blood, a separate category, is a bit of a weird one. Of course, we all have blood, but in this case, it is meant in terms of blood quality. In Chinese culture, blood quality is measured by the nourishment circulating in our bodies. Eating certain foods can improve that quality.

Essence or Jing is stored in the kidneys and is responsible for growth and development. Although it is partially inherited from parents, it is also heavily influenced by lifestyle, eating, and drinking habits. This shows a belief system of eating completely centered around restoring energy through food.

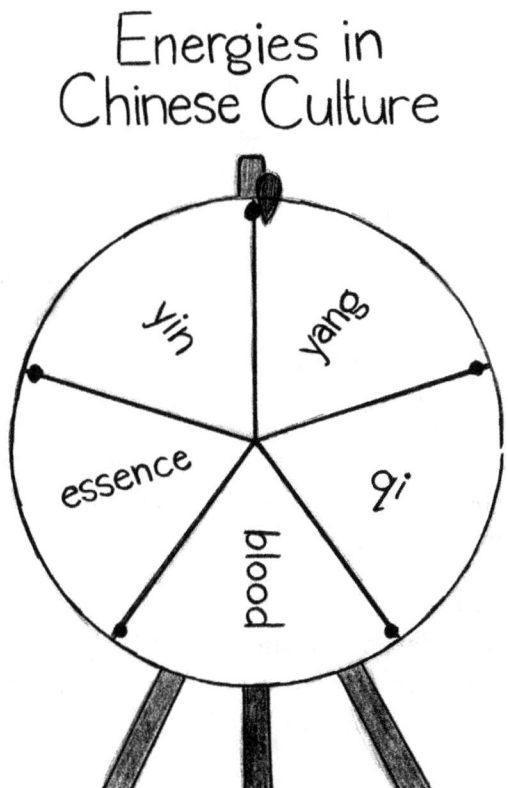

The general considerations of eating well in Chinese culture revolve around joy, having a positive attitude toward food, and accepting food lovingly (not categorizing it as good or bad), and the use of relaxation.

This mainly pertains to their beliefs to not mix food and work (which is, of course, not fully possible nowadays), but in their culture, they stress taking several deep breaths before eating and not eating with crossed legs or sitting hunched as it compresses digestive organs and hinders their passage.

The Chinese also believe chewing well is important to lessen the work of digestive organs. They recommend you stop eating even before you feel full. This again lessens the load on the digestive system. (These cultural practices are amazing and should be taught and embraced everywhere!)

In oriental medicine, every organ falls under a particular element. The digestive system belongs to Earth, the provider of nourishment and support. It also encourages the choosing of foods and trusting your bodily instincts as its connection to Earth has a deeper level of knowing.

This means that if you feel you are craving something salty, perhaps it is because your electrolyte balance is low and eating some lightly salted nuts or olives would replenish your body's levels (rather than reaching for a deep-fried bag of chips).

Oriental medicine also differs from Western medicine as food is usually explained as containing amounts of protein, fat, and carbohydrates (hell, I even did that in this book).

In the East, food is described as having a warming or cooling nature, possessing a certain flavor, or acting on the body in a certain way. The warming and cooling effect does not pertain to the temperature of the food but rather to the measure of its effect on the body.

For example, cooling foods direct energy inward and down. Warming foods move energy upward and outward from the core, speeding us up. Different types of foods hold warm or cool properties.

For example, high-water-content foods like cucumbers and melons have cooling effects on the body (hence why they grow in spring and summer, when the weather is hot), whereas root vegetables and aromatic spices have warmer effects on the body (they are typically grown in the fall and winter). You see, Mother Nature has thought of everything.

Every flavor is also associated with an element and is said to enter one organ in their culture. The salty flavor is associated with water and enters the kidney. It drives food toward the root of the body and regulates moisture balance within. It stimulates the digestive function and improves concentration.

A sour flavor is associated with wood and enters the liver, where it stimulates contraction and absorption. It counteracts fatty foods and lowers the acidity of the intestines. A bitter taste is known to be associated with fire, and it enters the heart. It betters appetite and stimulates digestion.

The sweet flavor (my favorite) is associated with the Earth and our digestive system. There are two categories: full sweet and empty sweet. Full sweet refers to foods like meat, legumes, nuts, dairy, and starchy vegetables that strengthen us. Empty sweet foods are added sweeteners with no nutritional input.

The last flavor is the pungent flavor, which belongs to the metal family and enters the lungs. It promotes the circulation of energy and blood, stimulates digestion, and helps break through mucus.

Flavor	Element	Function
Salty	Water	Enters the kidney and regulates moisture balance, stimulates digestion, and improves concentration.
Sour	Wood	Enters the liver and stimulates contraction and absorption. It also counteracts fatty foods and lowers the acidity of the intestines.
Bitter	Fire	Enters the heart, betters appetite, and stimulates digestion.
Sweet	Earth	Enters digestive system/spleen. Full sweet refers to whole foods, whereas empty sweet is added sugars.
Pungent	Metal	Enters the lungs and promotes the circulation of blood and energy, stimulates digestion, and helps break through mucus.

I know this can all be very confusing. This is a vague description of how the oriental beliefs toward food and energetics influence the body and the food choices they make.

They eat based on their energy sources, organs, and flavors to seek out the highest vibration of foods for their particular ailments or bodily needs. They firmly believe that when we are out of balance, we develop a craving for a certain flavor or food that attempts to correct the imbalance.

This speaks to how our bodies are intuitive and how foods hold energy and medicine-like qualities. We have an inner knowing, and it's time we got back in touch with it to lift ourselves from the low-energy fog plaguing our current society.

So often in Western culture, we are taught from a young age about "good" and "bad" foods. This can create restriction and guilt when we give into our temptations and can set up a pattern of disordered eating. Take a note from oriental medicine and start adapting a more inclusive mindset to food (and I mean whole foods that don't come in a package)!

Energetics Tips

Increase your Intake of High Vibrational Foods

This goes without saying, but when I say to increase your intake of high-vibrational foods, I am also hinting for you to decrease your intake of low-vibrational foods.

The first thing I tell my clients is to stop keeping it in the house. Stop buying the stuff, throw it out, or better yet, give it to your arch-nemesis as a gift! (Joking, don't do that.) When it is out of sight, it is out of mind.

Of course, from time to time, go for it and splurge! Enjoy some chips or chocolate or ice cream. But in moderation. In the meantime, up your intake of vegetables and fruits. You will see huge differences in your energy levels, brain fog, and fatigue.

Swap your usual snacks that might have consisted before of solely processed foods for chopped veggies and homemade hummus or a fruit salad.

If you are a busy person, working parent, or just can't be bothered in the kitchen, I find it most useful to chop up the veggies and fruits after grocery shopping, wash them properly, and store them in containers for the week so you can just grab and go.

You can also place more emphasis on adding vegetables to your meals as another way to up those vibrations. Some of the best vibrational foods include kale, berries, sweet potatoes, apples, avocados, pomegranates, ginger, and herbs. Experiment and go for it!

Eat in a Social Setting

Feel like you've heard this one before? You have. We've got some repetition going on. What's good for your gut-brain connection is also going to elevate the vibration you are receiving while eating.

Ensuring positive emotions are created while eating is a surefire way to enhance the vibration, whereas the opposite is true when eating in a negative state.

Eating together will foster positive memories, and it is a good habit to build while your kids are growing up. Try to encourage them to put devices away and really tune into that family time and enjoy the amazing food together, no matter how much they beg for one more game or text being sent.

Try Holistic Methods of Healing Rather Than Conventional Methods

Rather than seeking out those pills for your constipation, acne, GI disorder, or difficulty sleeping etc., etc., etc., why don't you try using your food to heal yourself? I know. I know. I was also a bit skeptical at first, too.

But now that you have learned about the vibrational qualities of different foods, you can get a better sense of what eating right and eating certain types of foods can do to help your body restore and repair itself.

The next time you feel constipated, go to the shop and get some apples, dates, papayas, aloe vera, and prunes. Rather than popping a laxative, you can 100% heal your gut by using the medicine Mother Nature gave us.

Running because you've got a case of the shits? Add some pear, red clover, and kiwi to your diet, and that should do the trick. (Also, be sure to rehydrate with filtered water as diarrhea leaves the body seriously dehydrated.)

Acupuncture is another alternative healing method derived from Eastern medicine practices. It has shown tremendous results in helping digestive disorders.

Having trouble sleeping? Try eating a mango before bed as mango is known to calm neuroreceptors in the brain. Switch off your devices 30 minutes before bed and either meditate, read, or do both to calm yourself. Breathing exercises are another great tool for this.

I recommend you do some research as to different alternative healing methods that can help whatever ailment you may be facing and try those before seeking out conventional methods, as they usually come with side effects and the vicious cycle of getting more pills to fix those. Get off the hamster wheel and take matters into your own hands.

Energetics Themes

Maybe you still think this topic is a bit hula-la, a bit out of the box. But there is the science to back it up. And even if you still don't believe me, I encourage you to experiment with it.

It is proven that everything gives off a vibrational frequency, and living beings give off higher frequencies than dead objects and foods. So, try to swap out processed foods and eat higher-frequency foods listed above. Document how you feel every day in a wellness journey and note your sensations.

Do you feel as tired as usual? Do you need as much food or caffeine aids to get through your day? Are you more productive?

You can really change your health and many other aspects of your life, like your relationships, your work output and productivity, as well as your financial and mental health through increasing the vibrational frequency of your foods.

I also encourage you to experiment with using alternative healing practices for any ailments you may be experiencing and note when and in which ways you start to feel better.

Drugs are not the solution for everything, however, you should still speak with your doctor and registered health coach to make a joint decision on which practices are best for you. Perhaps there are better ways you can heal that don't come with added side effects.

I am a firm believer that illnesses and infections are problems, and the solutions were created in Mother Nature for us to find and use, much like the beliefs shared in oriental medicine. These beliefs are extensive and exciting, and they truly deserve their own book, but it is fascinating to see how their healing patterns start first on their plate to nourish inside-out.

It is also interesting how the Orient contains the largest number of blue zones (people who live past 100 or centurions as they call them), and their eating and healing habits play a huge role in these findings. They are definitely onto something.

CHAPTER 6

A WHOLE NEW WORLD

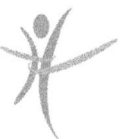

*"The only person you are destined to become
is the person you decide to be."*

—Ralph Waldo Emerson

Yes, I really did just use a line from *The Little Mermaid*. But that's what these discoveries and wealth of information gave me: a whole new world. It was a world where everything made sense, and what sat on the plate in front of me had the power to heal or hurt me, and I knew which one I would prefer.

This knowledge gave me the freedom to make my own choices regarding nutrition based on what worked for me. I stress that again. What worked for me! I really hate when TikTok or Instagram health influencers tell you not to eat this food or that food, or to simply count calories, or whatever lame-o advice they were once given.

Nutrition is so bio-individual. It is unique to me and unique to you. My hope throughout this book is to emphasize the bodily processes that go on inside of all of us. From there, I made recommendations not so much about what to take away from your plate but tips and tricks on how to eat those foods without disrupting bodily processes.

After all, if you want to eat your mama's pancakes for breakfast that remind you of your childhood, who in the hell am I to tell you that you can't?! Actually, that probably brings you a sense of relaxation and calms your stressors to help your body heal. (Just remember everything in moderation around a healthy diet, and probably try to have some apple cider vinegar before to calm your glucose reaction.)

Fad diets are not lifestyles. They are often quick (and sometimes painful) ways to lose weight, but they truly pay no caution to your health or how you feel. These two things are vital in designing a diet lifestyle program.

Keto, juicing, calorie counting, restrictive diets and shake diets are not the way if you can't sustain it for long periods of time. Get yourself a lifestyle that you feel great on and want to commit to for the rest of your life.

This is the first thing we focus on with my clients. When doing their health history consultation and seeing if we are a good fit for one another, I truly get a sense of the person—their stressors, their relationships, their careers, their activity, their diets, of course, and even their childhood upbringing. We work to design a program that fits their unique needs and that also encompasses tools and ways to heal their personal lives, which might have impactful consequences on their physical health.

The success rates we have seen are amazing, and I truly hope you one day, or perhaps you already do, feel this way! With all of my clients, however, I do advise one of the core principles highlighted in this book: to stray away from processed foods with all the added salt, sugar, and fat and get back to the roots of nutrition, whole foods. I guarantee that by making this small change, your health will drastically improve. If you feel you need a more hands-on approach and advice, be sure to check the end of the book, where I have a little surprise for you!

Our glucose discussion illustrated the importance of managing blood sugar levels and how certain practices can minimize glucose and insulin spikes without eliminating or restricting any foods! These hacks have served me and many others in reaching their goals and still eating the foods they love.

We learned about the four different types of sugars—starch, fructose, sucrose, and fiber—and the different ways they are metabolized in the body. The goal outlined by the American Diabetes Association was not to increase your glucose levels by 30mg/dL after eating, or in more simpler terms, maintain a flatter glucose and insulin curve.

The issue nowadays is that a lot of different foods (namely processed ones) contain large amounts of sugar, and our glucose levels have become dangerous, fluctuating to high levels after eating. This is then stored in the liver and fat stores and sets someone up for nonalcoholic fatty liver disease and puts them at risk for heart disease, type 2 diabetes, cognitive decline, and aging via glycation.

If your checklist from the glucose chapter contained a lot of ticked boxes, I recommend you try taking several of the tips I mentioned and also ask your doctor for a glucose monitor to track your blood sugar levels, and go through strategies to get those curves under control.

Our hormone topic was kicked off by outlining the five groups in which our hormones deal: the blood sugar group, the stress group, the metabolic group, the elimination group, and the reproductive group. Here, we could already see some overlap. When our blood sugar levels are steadier, it leads to happier and healthier hormones. Hmm … interesting. Almost as if our systems are interconnected or something (which I hope you now know just how much they are)!

Furthering our hormones wrap-up, we discussed how these messenger molecules function with our endocrine system. They regulate our energy levels, our physical and mental activity, and mood, setting our body temperature, metabolizing food, and determining fertility.

We also touched on the various roles our glands play and how they communicate with the brain based on hormone concentrations. Endocrine disruptors were then outlined with a major point being made about the effect of stress and hormones being added to many foods we eat on a daily basis, namely in dairy and meat products.

Not only does this set us up for hormonal imbalances, but it also throws off our other bodily systems and causes a ripple effect of issues, and yet it is approved by governing food bodies. Interesting. Another issue to tackle for another day.

The gut-brain connection was detailed at length, from the role the gut microbes play to the enteric nervous system to the vagus nerve. This was discussed to highlight the impact of emotions on our decisions and bodily processes.

Emotions can inhibit the digestive system, or they can speed it up based on the situation at hand. It is insane that automatic bodily processes can be interrupted by the sheer reaction from a stressful situation!

We explored how emotions and emotional connections to food can set up emotional eating patterns and how, on the contrary, positive memories attached to foods can heal relationships with food as a whole. The appetite process in the brain was further detailed to show how marketing campaigns and food restrictions can also affect this fragile process.

Lastly, we detailed the topic of energetics. I tried to get you on more of a spiritual and scientifically proven plan to show you how we are all forms of energy and that the foods we choose to eat are also forms of energy. Their vibrational frequency has an enormous impact on the level of frequency at which we operate and the electromagnetic energy received.

We pointed out that nutrient-dense whole foods have a higher electromagnetic energy and that it positively impacts energy levels as opposed to their processed, "dead" food counterparts.

Healing naturally was also briefly touched on but was just included as an eye-opener to different types of medicine; however, further explanation and research must be conducted by you and your health coach to see which option or foods are right for you.

Oriental eating patterns were shown to also demonstrate that food is regarded as a healing property, and perhaps some of those beliefs you read truly touched you and inspired you to adopt those practices. If so, then I am definitely a happy camper.

After relaying the main points from this book, I will do as I promised. I will tie in all of the main tips from each section of this book (as many have overlapped) and share with you the main practices I urge you to try to benefit not one but *all* your bodily systems and organs, leading you on the road to a healthier and happier food journey.

1. Eat more whole foods and less processed ones.

I mean, this was obvious. If you haven't caught on to this trend by now, then I suggest that you go back and reread.

Whole foods are not only more nutrient-dense, but they also contain the fiber necessary to regulate your blood sugar levels, the nutrients to soothe those stressed hormones and nourish your gut microbes, and the high vibration frequency to get your energetics up.

I suggest you try to crowd out your processed foods by simply adding more whole foods to your diet. Eventually, there will be no place for your old, processed staples, and you will have already felt major shifts in your health!

2. Listen to your body cues.

Although this was never explicitly said, I have hinted a heck of a lot about this. Your body is an all-knowing being. You know your body better than I or any other health professional will! So, all you need to do is listen to it.

That is why I hinted in the gut-brain chapter that certain cues can get missed or their sensitivity can weaken with the processed foods being eaten. Once you get back in tune with your gut, your cravings will start to direct you toward whole foods with vitamins that you need or might be missing.

Or, your intuition will direct you to get some extra sunlight (which is great for your hormones) or move your body. This idea of eating is one that we need to begin to adopt as food is always readily available, close by, and marketed effectively. Using the tips we have discussed will help your all-knowing power and direct you to the right foods for you.

3. Eating foods in the right order.

Remember how it goes? Fiber, proteins, and fats, and then carbs. Not only does this significantly flatten your glucose curve, but it also helps the hormones in your blood sugar group, as we covered. When your hormones are happy, your gut can digest effectively, and your stress and anxiety levels will plummet. Give this a try and see if you feel a difference in a couple of weeks!

4. Add vinegar before meals.

This hack has greatly helped me and my clients, so I urge you to try it. If you are like me and used to be scared of drinking apple cider vinegar, it really isn't so bad when diluted with water. The benefits far outweigh the taste. It slows the rate of glucose in your bloodstream and is so useful before carb-heavy meals. It will also greatly aid any weight goals you might have in mind. Again, this helps not only your glucose levels but also your hormones and gut health.

5. Opt for dairy-free alternatives and assess whether you might need to go gluten-free.

The reason I say go dairy-free is due to several of the reasons listed throughout the book. First, it is so heavily loaded with extra hormones yet, it is already a hormone liquid. It was designed to nourish baby calves, not humans!

It is known to be linked to severe bloating and acne symptoms due to the hormonal imbalances it creates. With the readily available dairy alternatives now in every coffee shop and grocery store, I'd say this one is pretty easy to convert.

Gluten sensitivities vary from person to person. If when you eat gluten, you feel very full afterward, bloated, and uncomfortable, I would say you have a gluten sensitivity and should opt for gluten-free alternatives. Experiment and see.

Both of these food intolerances will limit the inflammation in your gut and maintain a sensitive connection between your gut and your brain to keep emotions at bay, stress and anxiety down, and help that six-month pregnant bloating look vanish!

6. Try 1-2 days of your week without animal products, and instead, increase your intake of plant fiber.

Animal products are known to be very fatty and cause immediate low-grade inflammation in the body. If you can implement plant-based meals throughout your week or go a full day or two without using any animal products, your body will thank you!

Not only that, the environment will thank you for it! The deforestation rates in the Amazon will decrease if enough people partake, and there will be less strain on the livestock industry and therefore less cruelty involved in the animals' living conditions.

This can even potentially decrease the chances for harmful bacteria in animal products as better sanitary conditions can be undertaken with a lessened load.

Try opting for plant-based protein options such as adding nuts and grilled tofu to your salads, try a coconut or lentil curry for dinner, or, instead of buying iceberg lettuce, opt for leafy greens like spinach and romaine.

Doing this will benefit your hormones greatly, and also your gut microbes will absolutely love it! Give them some plant fiber; they are dying for it. You will experience increased energy from the high energetics that whole plant foods possess.

7. Take time in your day for yourself and destress.

A major reemerging theme throughout this book was the impact that stress had on our bodily processes. It is an endocrine disruptor, a flare for the gut-brain connection, and an inflammatory agent, and it decreases vibrational frequency.

Stress is linked to being a catalyst for cancer cells, and it is so vital to look after ourselves as a preventative measure. Try to add a yoga practice or two into your week and/or add breathing exercises to your morning. One that I love is called the 4-7-8 technique by Andrew Weil. Breathe in through your nose for 4 seconds, hold for 7, and release out through your mouth for 8 seconds for four breath cycles with your eyes closed.

Another great practice is to take a candlelit bubble bath with a cup of hot tea to warm and nourish your body. Or sit in nature and watch the sunset. Whatever your choice may be, it will nourish your soul and your body, and I encourage you to carve time out for these things, as they can sometimes do more for us than what is on our plate.

Of course, as you can see here, these are not all of the tips we have outlined in the book. If you tried to do all of them, you would probably drive yourself crazy!

Instead, I outlined the tips that touch all of the systems we have covered in this book to upgrade your health on all levels—without giving yourself a headache.

If there was one particular section and system you would like to focus on, then definitely write that down and implement those tips to take with you on your health journey. And just know that we are all human, and we aren't perfect.

Do what you can, and f*ck the rest.

CROSSING THE FINISH LINE

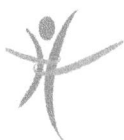

*"The first step toward getting somewhere is to decide
you're not going to stay where you are."*

– J.P. Morgan

Well, my friend, we've made it.

I truly am so grateful to you for picking up this book and making the decision to look after yourself. By implementing some of these practices, you will already be on your own health journey, if you have not already commenced one.

I want to remind you that you are different. You are unique. Your nutrition and various health practices will differ from others, and that is ok. That is how it should be. I wish someone had told me this long ago; however, it was a part of my journey to personally experience hardships so I could help you and many more like you.

I hope you take away knowledge, love, and kindness to yourself from my book. I am so freaking analytical that learning about my body and how it operates was essential to my healing journey, and odds are, if you've picked up this book, you are too.

I am deeply grateful to you and excited to be a part of your healing journey in some way. I hope I inspired a new way of thinking and kept it down-to-earth as I, too, have walked in your shoes.

Embrace this start of your health journey, and should you need further help and consultation, please don't hesitate to contact me, as I love to be in touch with my readers.

So, without further ado, I take my final bow, wave goodbye, and close the curtain … until next time.

ACKNOWLEDGMENTS

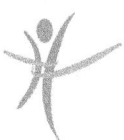

I would like to say a huge thank you to my parents, first and foremost, for investing in me, believing in me, and supporting me through accomplishing my dreams. They are the best role models I could ever have asked for in demonstrating what it means to help others, keep your head down, and work hard to create the life you've always wanted.

I also want to thank my boyfriend Dominik for reigniting the real me. For reminding me of who I am, my forgotten dreams, and for loving me unconditionally. Through the good and the bad I love you and am beyond grateful for you.

Huge thanks go to the coaches I have had throughout my dancing career and the team that helped build my mindset, dedication, and discipline and ultimately helped shape who I am today. The skills and mindset I have acquired through my many years of dancing are priceless, and I would do it all over again a million times over.

I would also like to extend my sincere gratitude and appreciation to the Institute of Integrative Nutrition for the beautiful knowledge, resources, and business support I have received. This education has helped my health journey, and it has helped me translate it into something I can use to help other women around the world. This information should be in the hands of every woman, and I hope this book brings that a step closer.

My sincere gratitude goes out to my wonderful team behind the making of this book and for helping me make this dream a reality; Lori Lynn, my incredible editor, Mary Rembert, my helpful proofreader, and of course Shanda Trofe, my amazing book designer. I also would like to thank Jaclyn Wong for her gorgeous graphics placed throughout the book, and my wonderful mentor and friend, Robyn Lee for her heartfelt foreword for my first book.

Lastly, I want to thank you. You have made it all the way through the book. You are the driver of your change and the creator of your life. I hope my book has helped you look at your body in a new light and helped shape your idea of health. I am so proud of your progress, and I hope to connect with you one day. If you enjoyed this book, don't hesitate to reach out on Instagram or TikTok. I would love to meet you! Thank you, you gorgeous, badass goddess!

APPENDIX

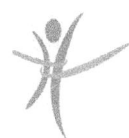

Bio-Individuality: a health practice catered to the belief that everyone's health needs are different and can change over a lifetime.

Bile: fluid that helps with digestion by breaking down fats into fatty acids, which are released by the liver and stored in the gallbladder.

Calorie: a unit of energy.

Calorie Counting: a health practice centered around tracking a desired number of calories taken in throughout the day.

Carbohydrate: one of the three important macros. Once your body breaks down carbs, it turns to sugar and is used by the body as energy.

Colon: commonly referred to as the bowel that is involved in the digestion process.

Detox Diet: short-term cleanses through the aid of vegetables, fruits, intermittent fasting, teas, and laxatives designed to rid the body of toxins.

Diet: the intake of calculated nutrition for health purposes.

Dopamine: a type of neurotransmitter and hormone that plays a role in memory, movement, pleasure, and motivation.

Endocrine System: a compilation of organs and glands responsible for reproduction, elimination, metabolism, blood sugar maintenance, and stress and mood.

Energetics: a principle of Chinese medicine that looks at how the energies of foods affect the body.

Enteric Nervous System: a large number of neurons designed to aid the gastrointestinal tract and its functions.

Esophagus: muscular tube that passes food and liquid from the throat to the stomach.

Fat: one of the three macros that helps give your body energy, protects energy, supports cell growth, keeps cholesterol and blood pressure under control, and helps your body absorb nutrients.

Fiber: a type of sugar that helps to regulate other sugars and hunger.

Fructose: a type of sugar naturally occurring in fruits.

Gallbladder: organ found beneath the liver that holds bile.

Glucose: a simple sugar.

Gluten: a type of protein found in wheat, rye, and barley that helps hold food together.

Gut-Brain Axis: the communication between the enteric nervous system and the gut.

Gut Microbes: microorganisms, including bacteria, fungi, and viruses, that live in the digestive tract.

Hormone: your body's chemical messenger.

Insulin: a type of hormone your pancreas makes that enables your body to use glucose for energy.

Intermittent Fasting: a health practice where fasting is performed for 12-16 hours before eating within a defined window.

Keto: a diet approach where solely proteins and fats are eaten to burn fat for fuel.

Liquid Diet: a diet approach where one, two, or three meals are swapped for a shake or juice.

Mineral: a naturally occurring element.

Monounsaturated Fat: fat molecules that have one unsaturated carbon bond. Olive oil is a prime example.

Neuropeptide Y: a peptide found in the brain that urges the body to eat carbohydrates.

Pancreas: an organ located inside the abdomen that creates digestive juices and hormones.

Polyunsaturated Fat: fat molecules that have more than one unsaturated carbon bond in the molecule (found in fatty fish, plant-based oils, seeds, and nuts).

Processed Food: any type of food that is changed from its natural state.

Protein: one of the three macros. Proteins form the building blocks of your cells and are comprised of one or more chains of amino acids.

Rectum: an organ responsible for collecting your bowel movements before expelling them.

Salt: sodium-chloride inorganic raw material.

Saturated Fat: a fat that is naturally solid at room temperature. Cheese, red meat, and butter have higher percentages of saturated fat. Coconut oil is one of the best types of saturated fat for your health.

Set Point Theory: the theory that states your body's weight is genetically predetermined, and when it falls below that point, your body will slow down its metabolism to adapt.

Starch: an organic chemical produced by all green plants that falls under the sugar category when metabolized in the body.

Sucrose: a sugar composed of fructose and glucose.

Sugar: a sweet substance obtained from plants and used in the food industry.

Trans Fat: also called partially hydrogenated oil, this is the worst type of fat for your health and occurs when liquid oils are turned into solids through a process called hydrogenation (examples are margarine and shortening).

Unsaturated Fat: this type of fat is liquid at room temperature and is further broken down into either polyunsaturated fat or monounsaturated fat.

Vagus Nerve: a nerve that aids in the communication between your gut and your brain.

Vitamin: organic compounds that cannot be synthesized by the body that are taken in to help with growth and nourishment.

Yin, Yang, Qi, Blood, and Essence: energetic beliefs in Oriental medicine with food practices undertaken to strengthen.

REFERENCES

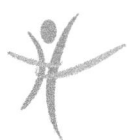

Beaman, A. (2021, May 1). *Girl Talk: Your Lymphatic System and Hormonal Imbalance*. CT Thermography. https://www.ctthermography.com/girl-talk-your-lymphatic-system-and-hormonal-imbalance.

The Brain-Gut Connection. Johns Hopkins Medicine. (2024, January 24). https://www.hopkinsmedicine.org/health/wellness-and-prevention/the-brain-gut-connection.

German, P. C. (2016, September 21). *Prenatal Stress Accelerates Growth and Inhibits the Motoric Development of Unborn Monkeys*. Phys Org. https://phys.org/news/2016-09-prenatal-stress-growth-inhibits-motoric.html.

Inchauspé, J. (2023). *Glucose Revolution: The Life-Changing Power of Balancing Your Blood Sugar*. Simon Element.

Leggett, D. (2005). *Helping Ourselves: A Guide to Traditional Chinese Food Energetics*. Meridian.

Mayer, E. A. (2018). *The Mind-Gut Connection: How the Hidden Conversation Within Our Bodies Impacts Our Mood, Our Choices, and Our Overall Health*. Harper Wave, an imprint of HarperCollins Publishers.

Psihoyos, Louie, director. *You Are What You Eat: A Twin Experiment*, Netflix, The Vogt Foundation, 2024, Accessed 2024.

Schroeder, B.O. *Fight Them or Feed Them: How the Intestinal Mucus Layer Manages the Gut Microbiota*. Gastroenterol Rep (Oxf). 2019 Feb;7(1):3-12. doi: 10.1093/gastro/goy052. Epub 2019 Feb 13. PMID: 30792861; PMCID: PMC6375348.

Tribole, E., & Resch, E. (2020). *Intuitive Eating: A Revolutionary Anti-Diet Approach*. St. Martin's Essentials.

Vitti, A. (2014). *WomanCode: Perfect Your Cycle, Amplify Your Fertility, Supercharge Your Sex Drive, and Become a Power Source*. HarperOne, an imprint of HarperCollins Publishers.

William, A. (2016). *Medical Medium Life-Changing Foods: Save Yourself and the Ones You Love with the Hidden Healing Powers of Fruits & Vegetables*. Hay House, Inc.

Ya'el, C. (2023, May 10). *Keto: It's Probably Not Right for You*. Science in the News. https://sitn.hms.harvard.edu/flash/2023/keto-its-probably-not-right-for-you/.

YouTube. (2016). *Dr. Valerie Hunt Energy Field Images*. Retrieved January 28, 2024, from https://youtu.be/9gJdC_f95A4?si=ipqvd0cgmZbpyjRD.

Zolfaghari, N. (2022, November 17). *Vibration in Foods and Moods*. Unspoken Nutrition. https://www.unspokennutrition.com/writingpieces/foods-moods-and-vibration.

Zoppi, L. (2022, December 5). *Sex Hormones in Meat and Dairy Products*. News Medical Life Sciences. https://www.news-medical.net/health/Sex-Hormones-in-Meat-and-Dairy-Products.aspx#:~:text=Growth%20hormones%20are%20a%20central,make%20animals%20cheaper%20to%20raise.

ABOUT THE AUTHOR

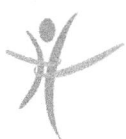

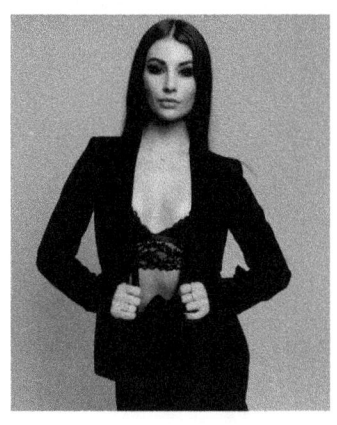

Morgana Lakatos-Hayward, a two-time Latin Dance World Champion and three-time Blackpool Champion, received her Health Coach Certification from the Institute for Integrative Nutrition.

After traveling the world competing in Latin dancing, experiencing body shaming and yo-yo dieting, Morgana finally found her way to food freedom. Now, she embraces bio-individuality and nonrestrictive lifestyle regimes as a certified health coach.

Her mission is to empower women to ditch diet culture and take control of their physical, mental, and spiritual health. On her podcast, *Listen to This When You're Done Dieting*, she combines her love of nutrition and physical activity as a health coach and her experience as a professional dancer to promote a holistic approach to living a healthy lifestyle.

You can find out more about Morgana and the health coach packages she offers at thisisntadiet.com.

YOUR FREE GIFT

As a thank you for reading this book, I'd like to offer you a FREE one-on-one consultation with me. Obviously, I can't do this for everyone, and I'm not sure how long I will be able to keep this offer going, but if the link below is active, you are in for a treat.

My initial one-on-one consults are comprehensive and last at least 30 minutes. During your free call, we'll address nutrition and movement and look closely at your mental and emotional health to ensure your life stressors are managed and that you have coping tools to use when stressful situations arise.

We'll discuss your symptoms, questions, and concerns before mapping out a plan that's targeted to your unique needs.

It's time to ditch diet culture (and the restriction and starvation that comes with it—which actually makes your body hold on to more fat!) and move toward health hacks that benefit your hormones, gut microbiome, and blood sugar.

You deserve to have the energy and stamina needed to accomplish your goals, live your ideal lifestyle, and look amazing doing it.

To get your FREE one-on-one consultation, call here:
http://thisisntadiet.com/pages/contact

www.ingramcontent.com/pod-product-compliance
Lightning Source LLC
Chambersburg PA
CBHW060505030426
42337CB00015B/1755